A Handbook of

Natural
Beauty

Other Books By The Same Author

— A Complete Handbook Of Nature Cure

— Diet Cure For Common Ailments

— Nature Cure For Children

— Naturopathy For Longevity

— Healing Through Natural Foods

— Indian Spices And Condiments As Natural Healers

— Foods That Heal

— Herbs That Heal

— Natural Home Remedies For Common Ailments

— Vitamins That Heal

— Conquering Diabetes Naturally

— Conquering Cancer Naturally

A Handbook of

Natural Beauty

Dr. H.K. Bakhru

JAICO PUBLISHING HOUSE

Mumbai • Delhi • Bangalore • Kolkata
Hyderabad • Chennai • Ahmedabad • Bhopal

Published by Jaico Publishing House
121 Mahatma Gandhi Road
Mumbai - 400 023
jaicopub@vsnl.com
www.jaicobooks.com

© Dr. H.K. Bakhru

A HANDBOOK OF NATURAL BEAUTY
ISBN 81-7224-370-7

First Jaico Impression: 1995
Seventh Jaico Impression: 2005

Printed by
Sanman & Co.
113, Shivshakti Ind. Estate, Marol Naka
Andheri (E), Mumbai - 400 059.

About the Author

Dr. H.K. Bakhru enjoys a countrywide reputation as an expert naturopath and a prolific writer. His well-researched articles on nature cure, health, nutrition and herbs appear regularly in various newspapers and magazines and they bear the stamp of authority.

A diploma holder in naturopathy, all his current 13 books on nature cure, nutrition and herbs titled, 'A Complete Handbook of Nature Cure', 'Diet Cure for Common Ailments', 'A Handbook of Natural Beauty', 'Nature Cure for Children,' 'Naturopathy for Longevity', 'Healing Through Natural Foods', 'Indian Spices and Condiments as Natural Healers', 'Foods That Heal', 'Herbs That Heal', 'Natural Home Remedies for Common Ailments', 'Vitamins that Heal', 'Conquering Diabetes Naturally' and 'Conquering Cancer Naturally' have been highly appreciated by the public and repeatedly reprinted. His first-named book has been awarded first prize in the category 'Primer on Naturopathy for Healthy Living' by the jury of judges at the 'Book Prize Award' scheme, organized by 'National Institute of Naturopathy', an autonomous body under Govt. of India, Ministry of Health.

Dr. Bakhru began his career on the Indian Railways, with a first class first postgraduate degree in History from Lucknow University in 1949. He retired in October 1984 as the Chief Public Relations Officer of the Central Railway in Mumbai, having to his credit 35 years of distinguished service in the Public Relations organisations of the Indian Railways and the Railway Board.

An associate member of the All India Alternative Medical Practitioner's Association and a member of the Nature Cure Practitioners' Guild in Mumbai, Dr. Bakhru has extensively studied herbs and natural methods of treating diseases. He has been honoured with 'Lifetime Achievement Award', 'Gem of Alternative Medicines' award and a gold medal in Diet Therapy by the Indian Board of Alternative Medicines, Kolkata, in recognition of his dedication and outstanding contributions in the field of

Alternative Medicines. The Board, which is affiliated with the Open International University for Complementary Medicines, established under World Health Organisation and recognised by the United Nations Peace University, has also appointed him as its Honorary Advisor. Dr. Bakhru has also been honoured by Nature Cure Practitioners' Guild, Mumbai with Nature Cure Appreciation Award for his services to Naturopathy.

Dr. Bakhru has founded a registered Public Charitable Trust, known as D.H. Bakhru Foundation, for help to the poor and needy. He has been donating Rs. 25,000 every year to this trust from his income as writer and author.

Preface

I firmly believe that true beauty, like good health, comes from within. What we eat has a profound effect on our health and appearance. This conviction prompted me to write a series of articles on various aspects of natural beauty and natural methods of treating beauty problems. These articles were published in many well-known magazines like Body and Beauty Care, Femina, Eve's Weekly, Mirror and Fitness.

The response of the readers, especially women readers, was overwhelming. Many of them benefitted greatly from my advice and succeeded in overcoming their beauty problems, especially acne and skin blemishes, premature greying of hair, falling of hair and patchy baldness. This encouraged me to make extensive studies of the subject and to compile the information in the form of a book. I have made a sincere endeavour to cover all aspects of beauty and prescribed methods for treating various problems connected therewith in a natural way. I have also dealt with a wide range of natural aids and their application in improving looks and apprearance.

There is a growing awareness at present that the cosmetics based on various kinds of chemicals are harming the users instead of benefitting them. More and more people are now discarding them in favour of beauty aids and preparations based on natural foods and herbs. I hope this book will contribute greatly to this growing trend towards natural beauty and provide a useful guide to every day beauty treatment.

Dr. H. K. Bakhru

A HANDBOOK OF NATURAL BEAUTY

CONTENTS

CHAPTER 1

INTRODUCTION

Natural beauty is a rare quality. It is a reflection of inward health and cannot be substituted by any amount of beauty aids. If you are not in perfect good health, both physically and mentally, your skin and hair will look dull and lifeless. Similarly, if you are not scrupulously clean no cream or lotion, however exclusive and expensive, will help improve your appearance. A healthy body and a happy state of mind are thus the basic elements of true beauty.

The chief attributes of natural beauty are clear skin, bright eyes, glossy hair and sparkling teeth as well as attractive features. While it is not possible to change one's features, a lot can be done for attaining other basic requirements of natural beauty.

One may spend huge amounts of money in an attempt to improve one's appearance with expensive cosmetics and beauty parlour treatments. But this will at best hide any imperfections and blemishes, but it can never give those basic attributes of natural beauty.

Women have always aspired for attractive appearance and youthful looks and searched for ways and means for their attainment. In ancient times, famous beauties attributed the longevity of their youthful skin tone to the use of herbal formulas. Then came the synthetic age with high pressure advertising, and the wonderful beautifying properties of natural substances were forgotten.

Women thought that chemical laboratories could solve all their beauty problems, that too in the shortest time.

Now the trend is the other way around. Recent years have seen a tremendous upsurge in the popularity of beauty products based on natural ingredients. This has lead to a revival of home-made cosmetics. Natural foods - fruits, vegetable, seeds, nuts, pulses and other natural substances are being increasingly used in the preparation of natural cosmetics. They not only enhance the beauty of the skin and hair but also possess curative properties.

Many are for this trend towards natural cosmetics. Every modern woman, like her ancient counterpart, wants lovely skin and glossy hair. But in her search for beauty, she has learnt that many commercial products that promise a glowing complexion and a healthy head of hair contain hormones, antibiotics, or other irritants that do more harm than good. Cosmetic reactions may appear as dryness, skin cracking, swelling, itchiness or as a rash.

Another reason for the growing interest in home preparations of natural beauty aids is the money-saving angle. Compared to the huge amounts women have been spending each year for commercial beauty products, natural substances cost very little. Women are also discovering that natural ingredients are often more effective.

INTRODUCTION

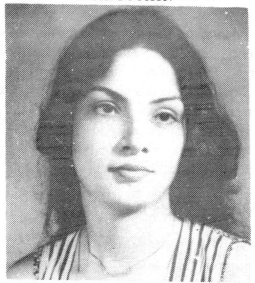

The chief attributes of natural beauty are clear skin, glossy hair and sparkling eyes.

The studies conducted by research scholars in the field of natural substances in recent years, have enabled us to use ingredients like almond, lemon, peach, turmeric, honey, rose, sandalwood and henna in preparations for the skin and hair. The products which form part of Indian heritage, like reetha, amla, brahmi, shikakai and others are also being used in the formulation of corrective cosmetics to treat many problems affecting the beauty of the skin and hair. Some of the natural substances even have preservative properties. This has helped to bottle natural cosmetics for longer periods, thereby eliminating the use of chemical preservatives.

The field of natural cosmetics is very vast. A knowledge about the properties and values of each of these will help us to incorporate them in the form of specific cosmetic preparations. The natural foods and herbs commonly used as beauty aids have been discussed at appropriate places in this book as well as separately in Chapters 16 and 17 titled 'Natural Foods As Beauty Aids' and 'Herbs As Beauty Aids'. The most important factor about natural ingredients is that they do not have adverse after reactions like those of chemical substances. As for the beneficial properties, they cannot be duplicated even in the most advanced laboratories.

CHAPTER 2

DIET FOR NATURAL BEAUTY

Just as diet and health are closely related, so also are diet and beauty. What we eat has a profound effect on our outward appearance as well as on our physical well-being. An ideal diet for improved looks is one which supplies adequate quantities of all the nutrients essential to health and beauty. The nutrients which are of particular importance for beauty and their main sources are mentioned herein :

(1) Vitamin A :

This vitamin is essential for healthy hair and eyes and for prevention and clearing of infections of the skin. It also counteracts dry skin, dandruff and wrinkle formation. Vitamin A is needed for healthy blood circulation which gives a glow to the skin. Lack of this vitamin is sometimes responsible for pimples or acne, visual fatigue and dull and dry hair. The main natural sources of this vitamin are cod liver oil, dairy products, carrots, green leafy vegetables, tomatoes, papaya and melon.

(2) Vitamin B Complex :

All the vitamins of B group are directly related to the health of the skin and hair. They are vital for youthful looks and for delaying greying of hair. These vitamins also counteract stress, which has adverse effects on one's appearance. A deficiency of B complex vitamins can lead to greasy hair, dandruff, dry skin, redness and irritation, wrinkles and poor hair growth or grey hair. Valuable natural sources of these vitamins are wheat and other whole grain cereals, pulses, nuts, green leafy vegetables, molasses, meat, and brewer's yeast.

(3) Vitamin C :

This vitamin is essential for the health of the hair, eyes and teeth, resistance to infection, healing of wounds and firm skin tissues. It reduces pigmentation and prevents bleeding of the gums. A deficiency may cause dry skin and thread veins. This vitamin is found in green vegetables, fresh fruits, specially citrus fruits, like lemon, orange and grapefruit, the Indian gooseberry (amla) and sprouted Bengal and green grams.

(4) Vitamin D:

This vitamin is essential for healthy teeth, bones and nails as well as for the assimilation of calcium and phosphorus. A deficiency can to dental decay. Valuable natural sources of vitamin D are rays of the sun, milk, butter, and sprouted seeds.

(5) Vitamin E :

This vitamin is one of the latest discoveries in the field of beauty. It is needed to prevent wrinkles, dry skin, brown age spots and dandruff. It helps to improve circulation and healing of scars. Whole wheat bread, whole grains, wheat germ, milk and raw or spouted seeds and nuts are the main natural sources of this vitamin.

(6) Protein :

Adequate protein is necessary for healthy hair, skin, teeth and nails and for firm skin tissues. Main natural sources are dairy products, nuts, pulses, wheat germ and brewer's yeast.

(7) Fats :

Fats are necessary to counteract dry skin and hair and for assimilation of fat-soluble vitamins. Main natural sources are butter, vegetable oils and nuts.

(8) Calcium and Phosphorus :

These two minerals work together for healthy teeth, hair, nails and bones. A deficiency of calcium in the diet can lead to tooth decay and recession of gums. The main dietary sources of calcium are milk products, whole wheat, leafy vegetables, orange and lemon. Phosphorus is found in abundance in cereals, pulses, nuts, fruit juices, milk and legumes.

(9) Water :

Water should be taken in large quantities, from six to eight glasses, throughout the day, except during meals. It gives the skin the necessary moisture and a dewy look. It clears the system of all toxins and keeps the blood free from impurities. Water also protects the skin against pimples. In case of insufficient intake of water, the body will draw on all its water reservoirs, including those of the skin, resulting in dehydration of the skin.

The nutrients mentioned above, translated in terms of food, represent a well balanced and correct diet which contains liberal quantities of (i) seeds, nuts and whole grains, (ii) vegetables and (iii) fruits. These foods have been aptly called basic food groups and a diet containing these is the optimum for the maintenance of good health and true beauty. This diet is described in brief as under

(i) Seeds, nuts and grains :

These are the most important and the most potent of all foods and contain all the essential nutrients needed for human growth. They contain the germ, the reproductive power which is of vital importance for the lives of human beings and their health. Millet, wheat, oats, barley, brown rice, beans and peas are all highly valuable in building health. All seeds, nuts, grains and legumes can be sprouted, and should be taken in that form as much as possible as they constitute live foods. There is an amazing increase in nutrients in sprouted foods when compared to their dried embryo. So potent are the sprouts that if one lives only on a mixture of these foods, one would have everything one needs for health and long lasting beauty. Sunflower seeds, pumpkin seeds, almonds, peanuts and soya beans contain complete proteins of high biological value.

Seeds, nuts and grains are excellent natural sources of essential unsaturated fatty acids necessary for health and true beauty. They are also good sources of lecithin and most of the B vitamins as well as vitamin C, which is perhaps the most important vitamin for the preservation of health and prevention of premature ageing. They are also rich sources of minerals and auxins, the natural substances that play an important role in the rejuvena-

8

tion of cells and prevention of premature ageing.

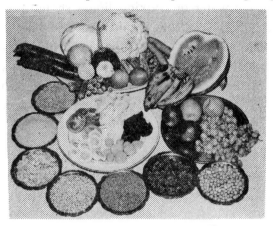

*A well-balanced diet is an important factor for ensuring good
health and natural beauty.*

(ii) Vegetables :

They are an extremely rich source of minerals, enzymes and vitamins. Faulty cooking and prolonged careless storage however, destroy these valuable nutrients. Most of the vegetables are therefore, best consumed in their natural raw state in the form of salads.

There are different kinds of vegetables. They may be edible roots, stems, leaves, fruits and seeds. Each group contributes to the diet in its own way. Fleshy roots have high energy value and are good sources of vitamin B. Seeds are relatively high in carbohydrates and proteins and yellow ones are rich in vitamin A. Leaves, stems and fruits are excellent sources of minerals, vitamins, water and roughage.

To prevent loss of nutrients in vegetables, it is advis-

9

able to steam or boil vegetables in their juices on a slow fire and the water or cooking liquid should not be drained off. No vegetable should be peeled unless it is so old that the peel is tough and unpalatable. In most root vegetables, the largest amount of minerals is directly under the skin and these are lost if vegetables are peeled. Soaking of vegetables should also be avoided if taste and nutritive value are to be preserved.

(iii) Fruits :

Like vegetables, fruits are an excellent source of minerals, vitamins and enzymes. They are easily digested and exercise a cleansing effect on the blood and digestive tract. They contain high alkalising properties, a high percentage of water and a low percentage of proteins and fats. Their organic acid and high sugar content have immediate refreshing effects. Apart from seasonal fresh fruits, dry fruits, such as raisins, prunes and figs, are also beneficial.

Fruits are at their best when eaten in the raw and ripe states. In cooking, they lose portions of the nutrient salts and carbohydrates. They are most beneficial when taken as a separate meal by themselves, preferably for breakfast in the morning. If it becomes necessary to take fruits with regular food, they should form a larger proportion of the meals. Fruits, however, make a better combination with milk than with meals. It is also advisable to take fruits in the form of juices.

The three basic health building foods mentioned above should be supplemented with certain special foods such as milk, vegetable oils, and honey. Milk is an excellent food. It is considered 'Nature's nearly perfect food.' The best way to have milk is in its soured form, that is yoghurt and cottage cheese. Soured milk is superior to sweet milk as it is in a pre-digested form and more easily assimilated. Yoghurt helps to maintain a healthy intestinal flora and prevents intestinal putrefaction and constipation. It is known for its health-building and beauty-enhancing properties.

High quality unrefined vegetable oils should be added to the diet. They are rich in unsaturated fatty acids, vitamins C and F and lecithin. The average daily amount should not exceed two tablespoons. Honey too, is an ideal food. It helps increase calcium retention in the system, prevents nutritional anaemia, besides being beneficial in kidney and liver disorders, colds, poor circulation, and complexion problems.

A diet of the three basic food groups, supplemented with the special foods mentioned above, will ensure a complete and adequate supply of all the vital nutrients needed for health, vitality and beauty. It is not necessary to include animal protein like egg, fish or meat in this basic diet, as animal protein, especially meat, always has a detrimental effect on the healing processes.

Sugar in any form is not good for health and beauty of the body. A high sugar intake is linked with diabetes and heart disease. One should, therefore cut down on sugar in all forms and use jaggery and other natural sweeteners like honey and molasses all of which provide valuable nutrients.

Apart from the quality of food which requires careful selection, the quantity of food we eat also has an important bearing on our appearance. Over-feeding puts pressure on the liver and renders the whole system inactive. It also adversely affects the circulations of blood. When the circulation is poor, the skin suffers from many disorders. Therefore, one should also limit the quantity of food one eats. At the same time, insufficient food intake can lead to many deficiencies, which may affect our health and looks.

Proper Cooking

Careful preparation and cooking of foods is also essential for health and beauty. Foods should be cooked in such a manner as to avoid unnecessary destruction of nutrients. It is healthier to roast or grill foods than to fry them and to cook at low temperatures for the shortest possible time. They should also be served immediately after cooking.

CHAPTER 3

SKIN : A MARVELLOUS MECHANISM

The skin, covering the human body, is a marvellous mechanism. It is the largest and one of the most intriguing organs of the body, accounting for 16 per cent of body weight. Its proper care is vital at any age. When one is young, it helps to prevent common teenage problems like greasy skin and acne. As one grows older, it is important to counteract the increasing dryness of the skin. One can have a beautiful skin at any age if one knows how to care for it.

Skin care usually refers to the face because this area, more than any other, needs care and attention. The face is constantly exposed to the elements, even in severe winter when the rest of the body is well wrapped. That is why the face is one of the first parts to show signs of ageing.

Functions : The skin performs many important functions. It forms a protective barrier against harmful bacteria and infections. Besides, it is a means of eliminating waste matter from the body in the form of excess water, toxins and carbondioxide. The skin also, as a sense organ, helps in regulating the body temperature, in respiration, and in the metabolic processes of the body.

The skin has three layers. These are the inner most layer known as the lower dermis, the middle layer called the dermis, and the outer layer known as the epidermis.

It is from the innermost layer that the various glands, including the oil and sweat glands, penetrate to the surface to eliminate waste matter. This inner layer is based on the fatty tissue of the lower dermis. It also acts as a cushion for the rest of the skin. It contains the finely distributed muscles of the skin which regulate body temperature.

The most important function of the middle layer of the skin is respiration. The countless tiny blood vessels, or capillaries end here in finely-drawn networks, from where they feed the outer skin layer. The tone of the skin is determined by the dermis.

The epidermis ranges in thickness from 1/20th of an inch on the palms and soles, to 1/200th of an inch on the face. It consists of several layers of cells. The outer layers of these cells are constantly shed as new layers replace them. This skin layer contains the nerve endlings. The oil and sweat glands open in the epidermis.

Types of Skin

The types of skin fall into four major categories : Normal, oily, dry, and combination.

An easy way to discover what type of skin one has, is to wipe the face with a dry tissue upon awakening in the morning. If there is oil on the tissue, the skin is a greasy type. If there is grease on the centre panel only, then it is a combination skin. If there is no grease on the tissue at all, it is either a dry skin or a normal skin. If the skin is left feeling stretched or too tight, shiny and parched, it is dry. If the skin feels smooth, supple and elastic, it is normal.

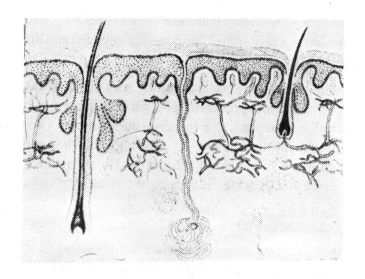

Diagram of the structure of the skin.

A brief description of these four types of skin is given below :

Normal Skin : This type of skin is soft, smooth, finely-textured and unblemished. There may be occassional pimples just before menstruation due to increased hormonal activity, which makes the sebaceous glands overactive. Acne is, however, never a problem for people with normal skin. This type of skin is neither oily, nor dry. It is beautiful, but it needs care if it is to last. Neglect can lead to signs of ageing and wrinkling. It should be cleaned daily with soap and water, and toned with something mild, like rose water.

Oily Skin : This type of skin is shiny, thick and dull coloured. It is prone to blackheads. In this type of skin, the oil producing sebaceous glands are overactive and produce more oil than is needed. The oil oozes and gives the skin a greasy shine. The pores are enlarged and the skin has a coarse look.

Oily skin needs special cleansing with plenty of hot water and soap to prevent the pores from being clogged. The flow of sebum or oil increases during adolescence and starts decreasing with age. During pregnancy and menopause, hormonal imbalances can also upset the oil balance and increase the activity of sebaceous glands.

Dry Skin : This type of skin is tightly drawn over bones and is often flaky. It lacks both sebum and moisture. It looks dull, especially on the cheeks and around the eyes. There may be tiny expression lines on these spots and at the corners of the mouth. In this type of skin, the oil glands do not supply enough lubrication to the skin which becomes dehydrated. Washing dry skin with soap and water not only removes grime but also the natural oils protecting the skin.

Dry skin needs plenty of thorough but gentle cleansing, regular stimulation with massage and generous quantities of oil and moisture. It also needs extra careful protection. A moisturiser increases the water content of the outer layers of the skin and gives it a soft, moist look.

Combination Skin : This type of skin has a greasy area, while the rest is dry or normal. The centre panel - forehead, nose and chin may be greasy and the cheeks dry. This type of skin is very common, and it should be treated as if it were two different types of skin, the dry part to be gently cleansed and regularly lubricated and the oily part deeply cleansed and toned. However, both the dry and greasy areas need moisturising.

CHAPTER 4

THE NATURAL WAY TO HEALTHY GLOWING SKIN

"All dress is fancy dress, is it not, except our natural skins?"

-- George Bernard Shaw

Healthy skin is an essential part of health and natural beauty. The skin of a healthy person should have a pink glow. Good skin is a reflection of inner health. However, sometimes we tend to ignore skin care until signs of neglect begin to show. As with health, prevention is easier than cure.

Causes of Unhealthy skin

One of the main causes of unhealthy skin is faulty diet. A child is born healthy and with a perfect complexion soft, smooth and flawless. It retains these for most of its early life. But as the child grows older, he gradually loses these attributes due to wrong feeding habits and other factors. Devitalised foods like white flour, refined sugar and all products made from them, tea, coffee, and soft drinks take away energy, bring about wrinkles, unattractive skin and premature old age.

Another important cause of unhealthy skin is the lack of healthy blood which not only adds a glow to the skin but also keeps it well-nourished, moist, and free from dryness and roughness.

Inadequate cleansing, which is responsible for many skin problems, is yet another important cause of unattractive skin. Do not be deceived if your skin looks clean. You will be amazed at how much hidden dirt appears on the cotton wool when you use a good cleanser. Proper cleansing not only removes all the dust, dirt and make-up, which accumulate during the day, but also stops the oil-secreting sebaceous glands from getting clogged.

Natural Care

Diet plays an important role in maintaining the health of the skin. Those with skin problems must have a vital diet consisting of foods which in combination would supply all the nutrients needed to build health, namely, protein, carbohydrates, fats, essential fatty acids and all the essential vitamins and minerals. Such a diet should consist of liberal quantities of seeds, nuts and grains, vegetables and fruits, supplemented by special protective foods like milk, vegetable oils, curd, honey and yeast.

All the nutrients are essential for a healthy skin. Thus for instance, if your skin is unusually dry and rough, or if you have blackheads and whiteheads, you are probably lacking sufficient vitamin A. Deficiencies in iron, iodine and the B Vitamins may also contribute to this condition. Adequate amounts of protein and vitamin C are also important. Both of these nutrients are needed before antibodies are produced to fight any infection and accelerate healing.

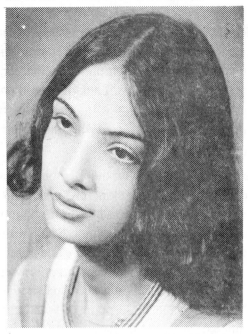

A healthy skin is an essential part of health and natural beauty.

The vitamins of the B group are important in producing beautiful skin. Vitamin B1 aids skin health by helping to keep the circulation normal. A mild lack of vitamin B2 or riboflavin, continued over a long time, causes brown pigmentation, or liver spots to appear on the skin. These ugly spots usually disappear if generous amounts of vitamin B2 are given over a period of six months. A quickly produced severe riboflavin deficiency results in oily skin and hair and small deposits of fat under the skin of the cheeks and forehead and behind the ears. A still more severe deficiency causes the skin under the nose and at the corners of the eyes and mouth to crack and become sore.

21

A lack of vitamin B6 or pyridoxine leads to dermatitis or eczema. A lack of niacin also causes an eczema type of skin eruption with brown pigmentation, largely on the face, forearms and legs. Lack of pantothenic acid, para-aminobenzoic acid, and biotin, causes types of eczema which can be corrected when these vitamins are generously added to the diet.

Since seven vitamins of the B group are directly related to the health of the skin, few foods can improve the skin so rapidly as those rich in these vitamins. Even the person whose skin seems smooth and healthy usually notices improvement in texture and glow, a week after adding two or more tablespoons of brewer's yeast to the daily diet. Persons with eczema should, for an entire month, take a tablespoon of yeast stirred into citrus juice or water after each meal, between meals, and before retiring. If the diet is adequate in all other respects, the eczema is usually cured in a month's time.

In case of unhealthy and unattractive skin due to anaemia, the condition can be corrected by dietetic treatment. Anaemia results from lack of protein, iodine, calcium, niacin, vitamin B6, vitamin B12, folic acid, cobalt, and copper as well as iron. In all anaemia, particularly pernicious anaemia, the vitamins of the B group should be generously supplied. Folic acid and vitamin B12 are especially important.

Natural Aids
Several natural aids have been found useful in promoting healthy and beautiful skin. One of the more important of these aids is the use of lime juice. Lime may be

squeezed in a glass of boiled whole milk and a teaspoon of glycerine may be added to it. It should be left for half an hour and then applied on the face, hands and feet before retiring at night. This application every night will help one to look young and beautiful. It will also help cure pimples.

The skin of the peach is useful in improving the complexion. 'A complexion like peaches' is a common expression. The inside of peach peelings should be gently massaged on the face every night for a few minutes. The moisture should not be rubbed off afterwards. This will cleanse the skin thoroughly and free the pores. It also has an astringent action and tightens the muscle of the face slightly, thus preventing sagging tissues.

The use of orange juice has also been found valuable for a glowing complexion. The fingers should be dipped in pure orange juice and the same applied liberally over the face, chin, neck, and forehead. Pimples and acne can be cured by anointing the eruptions at bed time with a paste made from the powdered sun dried pips of unripe oranges.

The juice of water-melon has been found useful in the removal of blemishes on the skin. A lotion can be prepared by grating and squeezing the juice of a small piece of water-melon. This lotion should be applied over the face and neck for fifteen minutes. Then wash with hot water and splash on cold water.

Tomato as an external application is a useful cosmetic. Its pulp should be applied liberally on the face and left on for an hour. Then wash off with warm water. Repeated daily, it will give you a good complexion and remove ugly-looking pimples in a short time.

Grated cucumber *(khira)*, applied over the face, eyes and neck for 15 to 20 minutes has been found effective as a beauty aid and is the best tonic for the skin of the face. Its regular use prevents pimples, blackheads, wrinkles, and dryness of the face.

The juice of amaranth *(chaulai-ka-saag)*, applied over the face with a pinch of turmeric *(haldi)* powder, bleaches the skin, prevents it from drying and wrinkling, cures pimples and makes one look fresh. If milk and lime juice is added to this juice and delicately massaged over the face and neck for half an hour and washed off with lukewarm water each night before going to bed, it acts as an effective skin tonic to increase and retain its beauty.

Application of fresh mint *(pudina)* juice over the face every night, cures pimples and prevents dryness of the skin. The juice can also be applied over eczema and contact dermatitis with beneficial results.

The seeds of radish *(mooli)* contain a bleaching substance and an emulsion of the seeds with water, applied over the face, will remove blackheads and freckles. It can also be applied with beneficial results in the treatment of ring-worm.

A paste of almonds *(badam)* with mild cream and fresh rosebud paste applied daily over the face is a very effective beauty aid. It softens and bleaches the skin and nourishes it with the choicest skin-food. Its regular application prevents early appearance of wrinkles, blackheads, dryness of the skin, pimples and keeps the face fresh.

Another effective natural aid for the beauty of the skin is the application of curd on the face every morning and washing it off after a few minutes with cold water. This will keep the complexion smooth, healthy and fresh. A mixture of curd and lemon juice is ideal for softening hands.

A paste of lentil (masoor dal) and curd, when applied as a mask, cleanses the skin and gives it a glow. When dried, it should be removed with fingertips and washed off with water. Adding a few drops of the juice of margosa (neem) leaves to this paste is very effective in dealing with pimples.

The flour of the unroasted Bengal gram (besan) is a very effective cleansing agent and its regular use, as a cosmetic, bleaches the skin. In allergic skin diseases like eczema, contact dermatitis and scabies, washing with this flour will be useful. The flour can also be used beneficially in the treatment of pimples. The flour should be mixed with curd to make a paste. This paste should be applied to the face. It should be washed off after sometime.

The flour of the green gram (mung) is an excellent detergent and can be used as a substitute for soap. It removes the dirt and does not cause any skin irritation. Its application over the face bleaches the colour and gives good complexion. Honey, olive oil and a mixture of turmeric and sandalwood *(chandan)* paste are all very effective in rejuvenating dry, parched skin.

Protection Against Sunlight

Excessive exposure to sun can lead to many serious consequences, including sun-induced premature ageing. The skin which is repeatedly exposed to sunlight becomes leathery, wrinkled and loose. It may also become dry and acquire yellowish brown hue with liver spots all over. The skin may become inflamed, which may contribute to the breakdown of other cells and tissues. Excessive exposure to sun can also lead to thickening of epidermis and enlargement of sebaceous glands in the face, ultimately resulting in acne and pimples. It is therefore essential to protect the skin from exposure to sun. This can be achieved by covering up and using a sunscreen with a high protection factor on the exposed parts. Even with these protective measures it will not be safe to stay in the sun for long periods.

CHAPTER 5

SKIN DISORDERS
AND THEIR NATURAL TREATMENT

There are certain skin disorders which cause a great deal of embarrassment at an age when people tend to be sensitive about their personal appearance. The more common of these disorders are acne, dermatitis and eczema. These disorders and the natural way to treat them are discussed in this chapter.

1. Acne

Acne is perhaps the most common chronic skin disorder. It is an inflammatory condition of the sebaceous glands and hair follicles usually found on the face, the neck, chest and shoulders. It is closely related to the disturbance in the hormones experienced at puberty. Nearly eight out of ten young people between the ages of 12 and 24 suffer from some degree of acne.

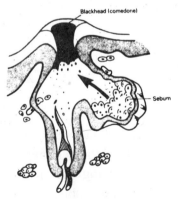

A blackhead is formed by sebum blocking a pore

Acne is characterised by the presence of comedones or blackheads, pimples, small superficial sebaceous cysts and scars. There are over half a dozen forms of acne. All of them are concerned with sebaceous glands or the glands connected with hair follicles. The most common form of acne is blackheads. The areas chiefly affected are the forehead, temples, cheeks and chin, the chest and back. In rare cases, almost the entire body may be covered with blackheads with extensive scarring.

All forms of acne have their origin in wrong feeding habits, such as irregular hours of eating, improper food, excess of starches, sugar and fatty foods. Chronic constipation is another cause of acne. If the bowels do not move properly, the waste matter is not eliminated as quickly as it should be and the blood stream becomes surcharged with toxic matter. The extra efforts of the skin to eliminate excess waste, result in acne and other forms of skin disorders. Yet another improtant cause of acne is a devitalised condition of the skin resulting from unhygienic living habits. Other causes of the disorder are excessive use of tea, coffee, animal fats, chocolate, alcohol or tobacco, strenuous studies, masturbation and sedentary habits which lead to indigestion and general debility.

Treatment

To begin with, the patient should resort to an all-fruit diet for about a week. In this regimen, there should be three meals a day, consisting of fresh juicy fruits such as apples, pears, grapes, pineapple, and peaches. During this period, a warm water enema should taken daily to cleanse the bowels and all other measures adopted to eradicate constipation.

After a week on the all-fruit diet, the patient can gradually adopt a well-balanced diet, with emphasis on raw foods, especially fresh fruits and vegetables, sprouted seeds, raw nuts and whole grain cereals. Further short periods on the all-fruit diet for three days or so may be necessary at a monthly interval till the condition of the skin improves.

The patient with acne should avoid meats, sugar, strong tea or coffee, condiments, pickles, fried foods, refined and procesed foods as well as soft drinks, candies, ice cream and products made with sugar and white flour. Starchy, protein and fatty foods should restricted.

As regards local treatment, hot fomentation should be applied to open up the pores and squeeze out the waste matter. Then rinse with cold water. Sun and air baths by exposing the whole body to the sun and air are highly beneficial. The healing packs of grated cucumber, oatmeal cooked in milk, and cooked, creamed carrots, used exernally, have been found to be effective.

The orange peel is valuable in the treatment of acne. The peel pounded well with water on a piece of stone should be applied to the affected areas. The lemon peel has also proved beneficial in removing pimples and acne. It should be applied regularly.

A teaspoon of coriander juice mixed with a pinch of turmeric powder is another effective home remedy for pimples and blackheads. The mixture should be applied to the face after thoroughly washing it every night before retiring.

Garlic has been used successfully in the treatment of acne. Pimples disappear without scars when rubbed with raw garlic several times a day. This even heals very persistent forms of acne suffered by some adults. The process is further helped by also taking the herb orally, to purify the bloodstream so as to secure a long-term clearance of the skin eruptions.

The juice of raw potatoes has also proved very valuable in clearing skin blemishes. This cleansing results from the high content of potassium, sulphur, phosphorus and chlorine in the potato. These elements are, however, of value only when the potato is raw as in this state they are composed of live organic atoms.

A hot Epsom salt bath twice a week will be highly beneficial in all cases of acne. This bath is prepared by dissolving one and a half kilo of Epsom salt to 60 litres of water having a temperature of about 100° F. The patient should remain in the bath from 25 to 35 minutes till he perspires freely. After the bath, he should cool off gradually.

2. Dermatitis

Dermatitis refers to an inflammation of the skin, both external and internal. It is characterised by redness, swelling, heat and pain or itching. Any part of the body may be affected by this disease. The exposed areas such as the eyelids, forearms, face and neck are more likely to be involved.

Substances which produce inflammation of the epidermis or dermatitis by mechanical or chemical disruption of the horny layer are called irritants. Degreasing agents like soaps, if used too frequently over a short time, will cause dryness, redness, fissuring and irritation of the skin in almost everyone.

The first symptom of dermatitis is erythema or redness. This is usually followed by swelling of the skin due to oedema (excessive fluid retention). Vesicles may appear thereafter. In case of their rupture, their bases exude serum. This condition is known as weeping dermatitis. Later, the serum dries up to form crusts. In some people the disease seems to come and go without making any great change in the skin itself.

Chemical substances usually give rise to dermatitis. They may reach the skin from outside or from inside through the bloodstream. About 100 different plants are known to be capable of causing dermatitis in susceptible persons. The onset is usually acute and begins an hour or two after contact. Dermatitis may be caused by external contact with mineral irritants. This includes most cases of industrial dermatitis which arise on the hands or forearms which actually come in contact with the irritant.

Certain drugs applied externally such as atropine, belladona, carbolic acid, iodine, mercury, penicillin, sulphonamides, sulphurs, tars and turpentine sometimes cause dermatitis. Other substances causing this disease include hair dyes, bleaches, skin tonics, nail polish, perfume, wool, silk, nylon, floor-wax and various detergents. Other causes of this disease are indiscretion in diet, deficiency of vitamin A and pantothenic acid, and nervous and emotional strains.

Treatment

As dermatitis may appear due to varied causes, treatment also varies accordingly. If, however, the trouble is constitutional arising from internal causes, the patient should commence the treatment by adopting an all-fruit diet for at least a week, as in the case of acne. After an exclusive fruit diet the patient may adopt a restricted diet for 10 days. In this regimen, breakfast may consist of orange or orange juice or grapefruit. Raw salad, consisting of vegetables in season, with raisins, figs, or dates may be taken for lunch. Dinner may consist of steamed vegetables such as spinach, cabbage, carrots, turnips, cauliflower along with a few nuts or fresh fruit. Milk puddings and desserts such as jellies, jam and pastries, all condiments, spices, white sugar and white flour and products made from them, tea, coffee, and other stimulating drinks should be avoided.

After the restricted diet, the patient should gradually embark upon a well-balanced diet, consisting of seeds, nuts and grains, vegetables and fruits. The emphasis should be on fresh fruits and raw vegetables. In case of a severe condition, the patient should undertake a fast having only fruit or vegetable juices for three to five days. This may be followed by a restricted diet for 10 to 15 days. Further fasts and a period of restricted diet at intervals may be adopted after the resumption of a normal diet.

The warm water enema should be used daily to cleanse the bowels during the first week of the treatment and thereafter as necessary. Epsom salt baths may be taken two or three times a week. The affected areas may also be bathed twice daily in hot water with Epsom salts. About 100 grams of Epsom salts should be added to a bowl of hot water for this purpose. A little olive oil should be applied after the Epsom salt bath.

The patient should avoid white sugar, refined carbo-hydrates, tea, coffee, and other denatured foods, and should make liberal use of fruit and vegetable juices. The combined juice of the apple, carrot, and celery is especially beneficial in the treatment of dermatitis. About 175 ml. each of these juices should be mixed to prepare 525 ml. of combined juice.

In case of trouble due to external causes, the most effective treatment consists of applying a mixture of baking soda (bicarbonate of soda) and olive oil. The alkaline sodium neutralises the poisonous acids formed in the sores and the oil keeps the skin in a softened condition.

The patient should undertake moderate physical exercise, preferably simple yoga asanas after the fast is completed and the restricted diet started. Exercise is one of the most valuable means for purifying the blood and for preventing toxaemia. The patient should also have adequate physical and mental rest and fresh air. He should avoid exposure to cold and adopt regular hours of eating and sleeping.

3. Eczema

Eczema refers to an inflammation of the skin which results in the formation of vesicles or pustules. It is the most common and most troublesome of all skin diseases. Eczema is essentially a constitutional disease, resulting from a toxic condition of the system. The disease covers a wide variety of forms, the majority of them being of a chronic variety.

Eczema in its acute form is indicated by redness and swelling of the skin, the formation of minute vesicles and severe heat. If the vesicles rupture, a raw, moist surface is formed. From this, a colourless discharge oozes, which forms skin crusts when it accumulates. The skin itches at all stages. In the wet stage, it may become infected with bacteria. Healing of the condition is effected by scratching in response to the irritation. Scratching not only spreads infection but also lengthens the stage of dryness and scaling.

Allergies play an important part in causing eczema. Some women get eczema on their hands due to an allergy to soap or detergents used to wash clothes or dishes. Some persons develop it around the fingers when they wear rings because of allergy to metals. Researchers at the University of Texas Health Science Centre at San Antonio, in a recent study of children with atropic eczema, found that 75 per cent were allergic to a number of foods. The most common triggers for sensitive persons are eggs, peanuts, chocolates, wheat, cow's milk, chicken and potato. The real cause of eczema, however, is the failure of the human system to excrete the poisons from the various orifices of the body. Other causes include faulty metabolism, constipation, nutritional deficiencies and stress.

Treatment

The best way to deal with eczema is to cleanse the bloodstream and the body. The treatment should start with a fast on orange juice and water from five to ten days, depending on the severity and duration of the trouble. This fasting will help to eliminate toxic waste from the body and lead to substantial improvement. In some cases, the condition may worsen in the beginning of the fast due to the increased elimination of waste matter through the skin. But as fasting continues, improvement will manifest itself.

After the juice fast, the patient may adopt an exclusive milk diet with beneficial results. In this regimen, he should take a quarter litre of milk every hour on the first day, every three quarters of an hour on the second day and every half and hour on the third day and onwards. The total quantity of milk consumed each day may be six litres. This exclusive milk diet may be continued for four to six weeks or longer, if necessary. Many cases of eczema have ben cured or greatly improved by using the milk diet, following the juice fast.

Fruits, salt-free raw or steamed vegetables with whole meal bread or chappatis may be taken after the exclusive milk diet. Carrot and musk melon are particularly beneficial. Cocunut oil may be used instead of ghee.

After a few days, curd and milk may be added to the diet. The patient may thereafter gradually embark upon a well-balanced diet consisting of three basic food groups namely seeds, nuts and grains, vegetables and fruits. The large proportion of the diet should consist of raw foods. Seeds and beans such as alfalfa, mung and soyabeans can be sprouted. This diet may be supplemented with cold-pressed vegetable oils, honey and yeast. Juice fasting may be repeated at intervals of two months or so, depending on the progress being made. In chronic and more difficult cases of eczema, the patient should fast at least once a week till he is cured.

The patient should avoid tea, coffee, alcoholic beverages and all condiments and highly flavoured dishes, as well as sugar, white flour products, denatured cereals like polished rice and pearled barley and tinned or bottled foods. The patient should eat only pure and wholesome foods.

Raw vegetable juices, especially carrot juice in combination with spinach juice, have proved highly beneficial in the treatment of eczema. The formula proportions considered helpful in this combination are carrot 300 ml. and spinach 200 ml. to make 500 ml. or half a litre of juice.

The patient should get as much fresh air as possible. Restrictive clothing should be avoided. Two or three litres of water should be taken daily and the patient must bathe twice or thrice a day. The skin, with the exception of the parts be affected with eczema, should be vigorously rubbed with the palms of the hands before taking a bath.

Coconut oil may be applied to the portions with eczema. It will help the skin to stay soft. Walking or jogging should be resorted to in order to activate the bowels. Sunbathing is also beneficial as it kills the harmful bacteria, and should be resorted to early in the morning, in the first light of dawn. A light mudpack applied over the sites of the eczema is also helpful. The pack should be applied for an hour at a time and should be repeated twice or thrice a day.

In cases of acute eczema, cold compress or cold, wet fomentations are beneficial. The affected part should be wrapped with a thick soft cloth. The cloth should be moistened with cold water (55°-60° F) every 15 to 30 minutes for two hours at a time. The bandage should be left intact, keeping the cloth cold. There may be intensification of itching or pain initially but this will soon subside. A cold compress may be applied twice daily for a week or so.

Steam baths may be taken two or three times a week with great advantage. They are especially valuable while on the exclusive milk diet. Neutral immersion baths lasting for 45 minutes to an hour, will also be helpful.

Certain home remedies have been found beneficial in the treatment of eczema. Of these, the use of musk melon is regarded as the most effective. In this mode of treatment, only musk melons are taken three times during the day for forty days or more.

Mangoes are considered another effective remedy for eczema. The pulp and skin of the fruit should be simmered in a cup of water for an hour. This should then be strained and applied as a lotion liberally to all effected areas, several times daily.

The green leaves of finger millet *(ragi)* are valuable in chronic eczema. The fresh juice of the leaves should be applied over the affected area. Certain liquids have also been found useful as washing lotions for cleansing the affected parts. These include water in which margosa *(neem)* leaves have been boiled, rice starch water obtained by decanting cooked rice and turmeric *(haldi)* water prepared by boiling water to which turmeric powder has been added.

CHAPTER 6

THE NATURAL WAY TO LOVELY
BRIGHT EYES

The eyes are a mirror of general health and the most expressive features of the face. Beautiful, bright eyes are a part of radiant health and the best asset one can have. They give a wonderful effect to one's personality. On the other hand, eyes are an indication of ill-health and a depressed state of mind. During illness, the eyes are the first to tell their story of pain.

Causes of Dull Eyes

The main causes of dull eyes are mental strain, faulty diet, and improper blood supply. Mental strain, resulting from overwork, worry, fear and anxiety puts a corresponding physical strain on the eyes and their muscles and nerves. Physical strain on the eyes may also be caused by reading in dim light or in glaring light, or reading in moving trains, buses or cars, watching too much television and films, and excessive reading. Dust, smoke and prolonged exposure to darkness are all harmful to the eyes and should be avoided.

Dull eyes are symptoms of a general toxaemic condition of the body mainly due to excessive intake of starch, sugar and protein. The muscles and blood vessels surrounding the eyes share in the clogging process taking place due to improper metabolism caused by an imbalanced and too concentrated diet.

For healthy and lively eyes, it is necessary that they are properly supplied with blood and nerve force. Any interference with the blood vessels or with the nerves of the eyes could result in lack-lustre eyes. The muscles covering the upper portion of the spine at the back of the neck are the main seat of mechanical intereference with the blood and nerve supply to the eyes.

Natural Care

The first important factor in restoring normal health and sparkle to the eyes is to loosen the strained and contracted muscles surrounding the eyes. The eye muscle and neck exercises mentioned below will help achieve this purpose. All these exercises should be performed while sitting in a comfortable position.

Eye Exercises

(i) Keep the head still and relaxed; gently move the eyes up and down six times. Repeat the same movement two or three times after a rest of two or three seconds in between. The eyes should move slowly and regularly as far down as possible and then as far up as possible.

(ii) Move the eyes six times from side to side, as far as possible, without any force or effort. Repeat two or three times.

(iii) Hold up the index finger of the right hand about eight inches in front of the eyes, then look from the finger to any other large object ten or more feet away- the door or window will do. Look from one to the other ten times. Do this exercise fairly rapidly.

(iv) Move the eyes gently and slowly round in a circle, then move them low in the reverse direction. Do this four times in all. Rest for two or three seconds and repeat the movements two or three times, using minimum effort.

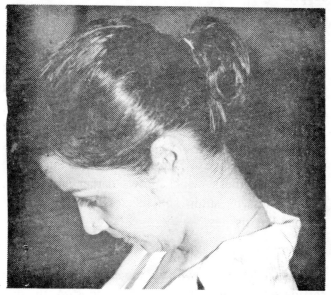

Neck exercises loosen contracted neck muscles and thereby improve blood supply to the head.

Neck Exercises

Rotate the neck (a) in cirlces and semi-circles, (b) move the shoulders anti-clockwise briskly, drawing them up as far as possible several times, (c) allow the head to drop forward and backward as far as possible, (d) turn the head to the right and left as far as possible several times. These exercises help to loosen contracted neck muscles which may restrict blood supply to the head.

Splashing

Splash plain, cold water several times on the closed eyes. Rub the closed lids briskly for a minute with a clean towel. This cools the eyes and increases blood supply.

Palming

Sit in a comfortable position in an armchair or on a settee and relax with your eyes closed. Cover the eyes with the palms, right palm over the right eye and the left palm over the left eye. Do not press on the eyes. Then, with your eyes completely covered in this manner, allow your elbows to drop on to your knees, keeping the knees fairly close together. While eyes are closed thus, try to imagine blackness, which grows darker and darker. Palming lessens strain and relaxes the eyes and its surrounding tissues.

Massage

Massaging the eyes with warm vegetable oil (olive or safflower) helps in getting a smoother look. As the skin around the eyes is very delicate, use gentle movements, without tugging. Start by running the third fintertip from your nose, under the eyebrow and in a circle around and under the eye and back to the nose. Repeat the movement using circular rotating actions, keeping them light and gentle.

Diet

Diet is of utmost importance for the health and beauty of the eyes. Natural, uncooked foods are the best diet.

These include fresh fruits such as oranges, apples, grapes, peaches, papaya and pomegranate; green vegetables like lettuce, cabbage, spinach, turnip tops; root vegetables like potatoes, turnips, carrots, onions and beetroots; nuts, dried fruits and dairy products.

Cereals are also necessary but they should be consumed sparingly. Genuine wholemeal bread is the best and most suitable. Jams, cakes, pastries, white sugar, white bread, tea and coffee, together with meat and fish, soon play havoc with the digestion and the body. Constipating or wind forming foods, alchohol and other intoxicating substances are also harmful and should be avoided.

Each of the essential nutrients needed by the body plays some part in the health and beauty of the eyes. The effect of vitamin A upon the eyes is, however, most pronounced. For normal and healthy eyes, liberal amount of vitamin A must be continuously supplied by the food. The valuable sources of this vitamin are cod liver oil, whole milk, curd, butter, egg yolk, pumpkin, carrots, green leafy vegetables, tomatoes, mango papaya, orange and melon.

If vitamin A is in short supply, the eyes may become sensitive to bright lights and a person may suffer from visual fatigue and a consequent feeling of tiredness. If a deficiency of this vitamin becomes severe, visual fatigue and sensitivity to light grow progressively more pronounced.

To keep the eyes normal, beautiful and bright, an adult should have at least 10,000 units of vitamin A daily.

Persons using their eyes for long hours or working either in extremely bright or in dim light require more of this vitamin that those who use their eyes for short hours. This vitamin is also essential to the health of certain tissues, known as mucous membranes, which line such body cavities as the tear ducts and tear glands. Healthy mucous membrane, or the normal flow of tears, determines the highlights, the sparkle, the charming play of shadows in the eyes.

Another vitamin necessary for visual health is riboflavin, or vitamin B2. Valuable natural sources of this vitamin are green leafy vegetable , milk, cheese, egg, citrus fruits, banana, tomato, brewer's yeast, almonds and sunflower seeds. Dull eyes and abnormal vision due to riboflavin deficiency can thus be found in almost any person who fails to eat these foods.

A healthy diet of milk, butter, fruits, green vegetables and proteins should be taken for the proper care of the eyes. Raw carrots, contain vitamins which help maintain the eyes in a healthy and bright condition. They should therefore be taken liberally.

Tears are believed to be beneficial to the eyes as they wash the eyes clean of dust and other particles. Medically, it is known that the enzyme lysozyme present in the lacrymal secretion is antibacterial and destroys pathogenic germs that enter the eyes. There are certain ways recommended to increase lachrymation like squeezing the rind of the orange or lime, crushing an onion close to the eyes and instilling a few drops of oil. Those who habituate their system to these practices from a

44

young age will benefit greatly. To start on these practices suddenly may not be easy.

Amongst the various natural substances, the use of castor oil is highly beneficial for the eyes. A few drops of this oil should be put daily in each eye. This causes increased lachrymation of the eyes for a while but leaves the eyes clean and cool. Regular massage of the scalp with castor oil decreases eye strain.

The herb nutmeg (jaiphal) exercises beneficial effect on the eyes. It is rich in fats and volatile oils. A paste of this herb made with milk may be appliied all around the eyes and over the eyelids. It will have a cooling effect.

Triphla, an ayurvedic preparation consisting of three myrobalans, namely, emblic myrobalan (amla), chebulic myrobalan (harad) and belleric myrobalan (bahera), is considered beneficial for long eyelashes and sparkling eyes. A teaspoon of this preparation should be soaked overnight in a cup of water. It should be poured through a clean muslin cloth and the eyes should be washed with it. The eyes should also be dabbed with the cloth for a minute. If a burning sensation is felt in the eyes, the water should be cooled in the refrigerator before use.

Cold tea can be used to brighten tired eyes. A cotton wool pad soaked in cold tea can be used as eye pads for this purpose.

Bathing the eyes in warm water, to which a little salt has been added, can brighten them. It also helps to relieve puffiness. A cotton wool pad dipped in a salt water solution, containing one tablespoon of salt in half a litre of water, can also be used as an eye pack for the same purpose.

Another important factor for the beauty of the eye is sleep. Without adequate sleep, the eyes can look puffy, bloodshot and even become encircled by dark shadows. At least seven hours of sleep is the average daily pattern. Whenever one misses out on sleep, it should be made good as soon as possible. As and when time permits, one should take a few minutes off to close the eyes and relax.

The eyes should also be proctected from long exposure to strong sunlight. The glare created by sunlight can harm the eyes. It will be advisable to wear sunglasses outdoors. It should, however, be insured that the quality of the glasses used is good.

CHAPTER 7

EYE PROBLEMS AND THEIR
NATURAL REMEDIES

Beautiful, sparkling eyes are the best asset one can have. They are an essential part of looking beautiful. They are also the most important medium of communication. By looking straight into one's eyes, a lot can be said about one's character, feelings and reactions.

The first essential for vibrant, sparkling eyes is that they should be clear and healthy. If the eyes ever get infected, or have any vision defects, an eye specialist should be consulted immediately for proper treatment. There are, however, some problems which are not so serious, but constitute unattractive highlights. These problems and their natural remedies are discussed here.

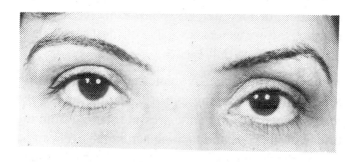

Beautiful, bright eyes are the best assets one can have.

1. Dark Circles

The skin around the eyes is very sensitive. It is thin in texture and wrinkles easily. The dark circles below the eyes can be caused by ill-health, such as anaemia or excessive menstruation during periods. In these cases, a doctor should be consulted. But sometimes they can be caused by simple factors like lack of sleep or a crash diet. Very often, the dark circles are a part of one's complexion. If dark circles are due to any of the causes other than heredity. The following remedies will prove useful:-

(i) Lie down on a board, raised at one end. Your head should be on the raised side. Now place cold cucumber slices over the closed eyelids. Relax for 10 to 15 minutes. Tea bags stored in the freezer can be used for the same purpose.

(ii) Eye Wash : If dark circles are accompanied by tired, red eyes, an eye wash should be used. This eye wash can be prepared by adding a tablespoon of Epsom salt to a cup of hot water. It should be followed by a few eye drops. Rose water also makes an ideal eye wash. It gives freshness to dull eyes.

(iii) Gentle Massage: A gentle massage can also help relieve tired and aching eyes. Using the tips of the middle fingers, exert gentle pressure starting from the bridge of the nose and tapping across the eyelids and back under the eyes half a dozen times. Then press quite hard on either side of the bridge of the nose close to the inner eye.

This is another common problem. It can be caused by ill-health, in which case an ophthalmologist should be consulted. If the puffiness occurs early in the morning, it may be due to water retention in the tissue. This happens as we lie prone at night. For quick relief, a large glass of hot water should be drunk on arising in the morning. This will stimulate the kidneys which tend to draw the fluid away from tissue. It can be made a daily routine if it works.

Another effective remedy for puffiness under the eyes or lids is potato. A raw potato should be grated and a teaspoon each, should be put in two square pieces of gauze to make an eye pad. The eye should be covered with these pads and left for 20 minutes. It should be followed with splashes of cold water. Another remedy for puffiness under the eyes is a fresh fig cut into halves and placed directly under the eyes. This should be applied lying down for 15 minutes. In summer, a grated fresh cucumber can replace the fig. Applying hot and then ice-cold tea bags alternatively to the eyes for 10 minutes also helps.

3. Lines and Wrinkles

These are inevitable, to some extent, with age. Some women, however, get tiny laughter lines quite early in life. These lines are caused by excessive dryness of the skin and loss of tone by tiny muscles around the eyes. A good moisturiser lavishly applied after cleansing and toning will take care of parched skin. A light-weight oil like safflower oil or corn oil is an ideal lubricant for eyes and areas around the eyes.

CHAPTER 8

THE NATURAL WAY TO
SPARKLING TEETH

The mouth is one of the materpieces of nature. With it, we express our thoughts and feelings and show affection. the process of digestion begins in the mouth and it thus sustains life.

The mouth is a delicate combination of skin, bone, muscles and teeth. The teeth are an amazing balance of form and function, aesthetic beauty and engineering. One can look one's best with a good smile, which is enhanced by good teeth.

Good teeth are thus an important part of one's health and appearance. Like the skeletal development, the appearance of the teeth and mouth is largely determined during the years of growth, depending on the amount of calcium, phosphorous and vitamin D in the diet.

Plaque

Proper cleaning is the most important step towards healthy and sparkling teeth. Ideally, teeth should be cleaned after every meal, but one thorough cleansing each day will be far better than any number of hurried brushings. A quick brushing is a waste of time. The teeth may appear clean, but they will still be coated with a layer of plaque, a sticky, transparent substance. It is invisible, but it can be felt as a fuzzy coating on the teeth. The accumulation of plaque can lead to gum inflamation and bleeding, which are early warning signs of gum disease.

Proper Cleaning

There are many theories on how best to clean the teeth. The consensus of dental opinion, however, seems to back using a circular motion with the brush, so as to ensure that all dental surfaces are cleaned. One should not be afraid to touch the gums with the brush, as this gentle stimulation improves the blood circulation in the gums.

Toothpaste is not in fact essential for the removal of plaque, although most people prefer to use it. It does help to keep the mouth fresh. The fluoride, which is now being added to an increasing number of pastes, also helps to strenghten the outer enamel and thus render it less susceptible to decay. It, however, has no effect on gum disease, which affects a very large number of people and is the main reason for adults losing their teeth.

Bad breath is not only unpleasant and embarasssing for the sufferer, but also for those with whom he or she comes into contact. With the efficient functioning of one's digestive juices, one is unlikely to suffer from bad breath. The breath can be freshened naturally be chewing fresh parsley or watercress, or by using rose water as a mouthwash. Commercial antiseptic mouthwashes should not be used as these are often too strong and can remove the protective fatty acids on the teeth and gum surfaces, leaving the enamel defenceless.

THE NATURAL WAY TO SPARKLING TEETH

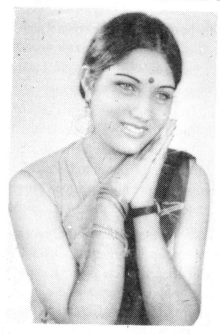

A woman looks her best with good smile which is enhanced by a set of good teeth.

Proper Diet

Diet plays a vital role in dental health. The condition of the teeth, after they are formed, depends upon the foods one eats from day to day. Dental decay, the destruction of the bone around the teeth, and infections of the gums, can be prevented with an appropriate diet. In fact, with the proper diet, the teeth and jaw-bones can be made harder and healthier as the years go by.

Probably the greatest curse and cause of tooth decay is the consumption of candy, soft drinks, pastries, refined carbohydrates and sugars, in all forms. Bacteria in the mouth break sugar down into acids, which combine with the calcium in the enamel, causing decay or erosion. It is therefore important to restrict one's sugar intake, and to ensure that the diet includes plenty of raw vegetables and wholemeal bread.

Whole foods are ideal. They are good for the teeth as the fibreless refined foods allow particles to accumulate on the teeth in a sticky mass, where they can do great harm. The gums need friction to keep them firm and whole foods also help remove plaque. They are therefore called 'detergent foods' by some dentists.

Whole foods, however, benefit the teeth only if they are free from sugar. Surgeon-Captain Cleave, the author of Saccharine Disease says, "It is perfectly true that refined carbohydrates are a prime cause of dental decay, but it does not necessarily follow that unrefined carbohydrates cannot be a cause. If they take a form of stale, coase, wholemeal bread and hard fruits and vegetables, no periodontal disease will follow their consumption".

In preventing tooth decay, what one eats is no doubt important, but equally important is when one eats. Frequent small snacks are very harmful to teeth, as they produce an acid medium in which the bacteria thrive. The number of times one eats sugar is one of the most important factors in determining the rate of decay. For this reason, it is better to eat sweets at the end of the meal rather than between meals.

Vitamins and Minerals
Every nutrient which builds health appears to play some role in the prevention of tooth decay. Much tooth

decay can be prevented if all persons, whether children or adults, obtained at least 1,000 units of vitamin D daily. Calcium is essential to maintain dental health. Adequate calcium can be obtained if sufficient milk is given daily to children and yoghurt is generously used by adults. A lack of calcium makes teeth susceptible to decay. The gums recede and the teeth often become loose and crooked, with ugly spaces showing between them.

The vitamins of the B group play an important role in preventing tooth decay. People who do not take adequate niacin have unclean mouths, heavily coated tongues, often foul breath and rapidly decaying teeth. Vitamin C helps to prevent decay by forming a strong foundation in the dentine, which contains the minerals. In short, all vitamins and minerals help to keep the teeth beautiful. A person susceptible to tooth decay should adopt a well-balanced diet containing all the essential nutrients.

Even though a person's teeth may be free from decay, unhealthy gums can lead to an unattractive appearance. Abnormalities of the gum tissue result from deficiencies and combinations of deficiencies. When vitamin C is under supplied, the gums bleed easily, recede, become infected, and pyorrhea may quickly set in. A person suffering from these abnormalities should include 300 or more milligrams of vitamin C daily in the diet. A glass of fresh citrus juice in the morning is of great value in keeping the gums pink and healthy. Lack of vitamin A can also lead to infections of the gums, causing them to look pale and unattractive. In such cases, more iron should be added to the diet.

Exercising Teeth and Gums

The teeth and gums, like other parts of the body, require exercise for maintaing them in healthy condition. This can be achieved by eating hard and fibrous foods. Wheat is especially valuable in the prevention and treatment of pyorrhea. It takes time to chew wheat chappaties, which are generally taken with other foods. This compels one to chew hard, not only providing the much-needed exercise for the teeth and gums but also helps the digestion process.

Chewing unripe guava is an excellent tonic for teeth and gums. It stops the bleeding from gums due to its styptic effect and richness in vitamin C. Chewing the leaves of the guava tree also helps prevent bleeding from the gums. A decoction of root bark can also be used as a mouthwash for swollen gums.

Preventing Decay Through Fruits

Tooth-decay can be prevented by regular consumption of apples, as they possess a mouth cleansing property. Dr. T.T. Hanks in his book Dental Survey says, "Apples have a mouth cleansing property that no other fruit possesses, and taken after meals, they have the same effect as a tooth brush in cleansing the teeth, with the added advantage that the acid content aside from its nutritive value, is of assistance in promoting the flow of saliva in the mouth, which is also beneficial to the teeth". The acid of the apple also exerts an antiseptic influence upon the germs present in the mouth and teeth when it is thoroughly chewed. Applies are thus regarded as natural preservers of teeth and should be taken regularly.

Grapes are very useful in preventing tooth-decay, too. The organic acids of grapes are strongly antiseptic. According to Johanna Brandt, "Every tooth may be loose in its socket and pus may be pouring from the gums, but after a few weeks on the exclusive grape diet, it will in time be found that the teeth are firmly set in the jaws and that every trace of pyorrhea poisoning has disappeared."

Lemon and lime also promote healthy teeth and gums, due to their high vitamin C content. They strengthen the gums and teeth and are very effective in preventing and curing acute inflammation of the gum margins.

Raw spinach juice is another valuable food remedy for the prevention and treatment of pyorrhea, because of its beneficial effects on the teeth and gums. This effect is greatly enhanced if the juice is taken in combination with carrot juice. A permanent aid for pyorrhea has been found in the use of natural raw foods and in drinking an ample quantity of carrot and spinach juice.

CHAPTER 9

KNOW YOUR HAIR

The hair is one of the most important factors which contribute to beauty and personal appearance. For its proper care, it is essential to have a basic knowledge of its structure. The hair is made up of keratin, a protein-based substance. This substance also forms finger and toe nails. Each hair consists of three layers. The central core, known as medulla, is made up of spongy tissues which may contain some colour pigment. The middle layer, known as the cortex, consists of long thin cells which give the hair its elasticity and colour. The outer layer, known as cuticle, consists of hundreds of tiny, overlapping scales.

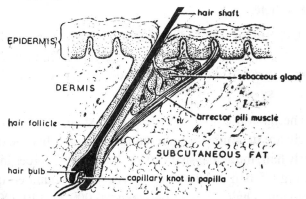

Skin, Showing A Hair Follicle
(A sebaceous gland is shown opening into the follicle.

Hair is formed in minute pockets in the skin, called

follicles. An upgrowth at the base of the follicle, called the papilla, actually produces hair, while a special group of cells turns amino acids into keratin. The rate of production of these protein 'building blocks' determines hair growth. The average growth rate is about 1.2 cm per month, growing fastest on women between the ages 15 and 30 years. The sebaceous gland which secretes the oil that gives healthy hair its natural shine is located half way along the hair follicle.

The follicles, which contain the hair roots, are fed by blood carrying nutrients. Good circulation is thus of utmost importance to healthy hair. It is the supply of nutrients which determines the health of the hair as it emerges from the scalp and continues to grow. Once hair leaves the follicle, it is in fact technically 'dead', but it grows because of continued tissue formation within the follicle.

A disturbance in the production of sebum by these glands can result in over dry or greasy hair. Thus, if the glands become blocked or are underactive, the hair will be greasy.

The natural colour of hair and its shape straight or curly are determined by hereditary factors. In case of curly hair, the actual shape of the hair follicle forces the emerging hair to develop waves. The number of individual hairs ranges between 90,000 to 140,000, depending on the natural hair colour. Blondes have the most hair since their hair is thinner than that of brunettes. Redheads have the least number of hairs, although theirs will often look more abundant since it is generally the thickest. The number of hair roots or the texture of the hair, cannot be changed except the natural changes which occur with age.

The life-span of a hair varies from several months to several years, depending on the scalp and hair conditions. The average life of a hair is five years. After that, the follicle from which the hair is growing begins to shrink and the hair remains static until it drops out or is brushed out and is replaced a few months later by a new hair. Although a large number of hairs may come out in a single day, it will not become thinner. The trouble starts when a new hair does not form in the follicle due to inadequate blood supply, or glandular or hormonal imbalance.

There are four types of hair -- normal, greasy, dry and greasy- dry. Normal hair is shiny yet not greasy, and fairly easy to manage. Greasy hair looks good for a day or two after shampooing but then quickly becomes lank. Dry hair is difficult to control after shampooing, looks dull and has ends that are dry and split. Greasy-dry hair is usually fairly long and the hair nearest the scalp is greasy while the ends are dry.

CHAPTER 10

THE NATURAL WAY TO GLOSSY HAIR

Lovely, shining hair is one of the greatest assets of a woman's beauty. It is considered a vital element of sex appeal. The most important factor for healthy condition of the hair is to ensure that the body is supplied with all the essential nutrients. The advice contained in chapter 2 on 'Diet for Natural Beauty' applies equally to hair.

There are, however, certain nutrients which are of particular importance to health of the hair. The vitamins of B group, especially pantothenic acid, influence hair growth, oil production and colour. An adequate supply of these vitamins is thus essential. Vitamins A and C also play an important role in the production of healthy hair, and vitamin E encourages hair growth by carrying oxygen to the hair roots. To ensure an adequate intake of the essential fatty acids, it is advisable to include two teaspoons of sunflower or safflower oil in the daily diet. Since the hair is made from keratin, the diet should include adequate quantities of protein in the form of dairy products, pulses and nuts. Of the minerals, zinc, copper, iron and iodine are essential to healthy hair. Copper is adequately available in food. Good sources of iron are liver, kidneys, whole grains, and molasses. The only foods that contain appreciable quantities of iodine are sea foods.

The hair, like the skin, is affected not only by diet and health, but also by tension. In a person who is tense, the muscles at the base of the neck are constricted, and this impedes the the flow of blood to the scalp, resulting in weak hair growth.

Hair Care

The care for the hair depends on its type. There are, however, certain basic guidelines which apply to all types.

It is a mistake to wash the hair too frequently. This is likely to do more harm than good. Shampoos may make hair clean, but at the same time they remove the natural oils and protective acid coating. A study at Cornell University found that shampooing created a loss of calcium, phosphorus, iron, and nitrogen from the hair. This came as a result of continued washing either with soap or commercial shampoos. It is therefore essential to use the type of shampoo that will do the least damage to the hair. The following tips regarding shampoo will be useful:

(i) Use shampoo only when absolutely necessary.

(ii) Avoid using hard water, or water containing chemicals including chlorine. Rain water is ideal.

(iii) Use a rinse after shampooing to undo the damage of the shampoo-vinegar or lemon juice may be used.

Brushing

Brushing the hair regularly is essential both to free it of dust, dead cells and tangles and to stimulate the scalp. A brush which has bristles with rounded tips is best, since it is less likely to scratch the scalp or tear and split the hair. A rubber cushioned brush is the easiest to clean, and is more flexible for gentle styling.

In case of short hair, it is advisable to use a brush with short, densely spaced bristles. For long hair, a vent angle brush, which has lots of space between the bristles, is better for getting the tangles out. Radial brushes, which have a completely circular base, are the best choice for styling curls while blow drying.

The choice of combs also depends on the type of hair. Wide-tooth combs are designed for very coarse or tightly curled hair. A fine toothed tail comb is used for lifting sections of hair, while blow drying, roller setting or for curling hair back into shape without upsetting the overall style. In case of an ordinary comb, a plastic one with rounded teeth is ideal. The larger end should be initially used to ease it through the hair, and the fine end to get a smooth, even finish.

The most effective way to brush the hair is to bend forward from the waist with the head down towards the ground, and brush from the nape of the neck forwards towards the forehead. Short hair can be brushed right from the roots to the ends in one stroke, but in case of long hair, two strokes should be used for the length of each hair, to avoid stretching it.

A scalp massage should be resorted just before or after brushing the hair. Like brushing this will stimulate the circulation, dislodge dirt and dandruff, and encourage hair growth. For a massage, fingers should be spread fan wise and slipped through the hair. With the thumbs pressed behind the ears, press down on the scalp with the fingertips. Now rotate the fingers so that they move the scalp over the bony structure of the head. You will feel your skin move and the scalp tingle. Move up an inch at a time until you have covered the whole head. It is a very simple procedure and takes only a few minutes to perform. The scalp should be massaged daily if time permits, or at least once a week.

Washing

The correct way to wash the hair is to use warm and not hot water, preferably from the shower. Once the hair is wet, a small quantity of shampoo should be applied, tipping it on the palm of the hand and rubbing the hands together. Shampoo should never be applied directly to the hair as this makes it difficult to get an even distribution. Work the shampoo gently but firmly all over the scalp using a circular motion. This method of massaging of the scalp encourages good circulation and ensures cleanliness of the hair. Continue to massage the shampoo in for several minutes, using the tips of the fingers rather than the nails.

A second application of shampoo is needed only if your hair is really dirty. After shampooing, give the hair a really good rinse, and go on rinsing it till the last trace of soap is removed.

Conditioning

A hair conditioner should be applied after the hair has been thoroughly cleansed. These products are especially helpful for long hair, where the overlapping scales which cover the outer layer of hair often get roughed up as it grows. A conditioner helps to smooth these scales down, and to give gleaming hair which is easier to comb and manage. Hair that is coloured, permed or exposed to the sun also benefits from a conditioner. Usually, dry hair should be conditioned once a week, normal hair once a fortnight, and greasy hair not more than once a month.

All conditioners are basically a combination of oils or waxes, detergents and emulsifiers, with optional extra ingredients, often incorporating herbal extracts with gentle plant and vegetable oils and essences. After conditioning, rinse your hair again, adding cider vinegar or lemon juice.

Drying and Styling

It is important that the hair should be dried correctly in a natural way. It can be easily damaged when wet. First of all the head should be wrapped in a clean towel for a few minutes to remove excess moisture. Rubbing with the towel should be avoided. When the hair is wet, a comb should be used as brushing will stretch and tear it.

The best way to dry the hair naturally is finger drying. If you want to use a hair dryer, always have it on the coolest setting, since heat dries out the hair. Most damage is done by over drying, so avoid holding the dryer over one area for too long, and stop drying your hair a few minutes before it feels completely dry. For the same reason, it is advisable not to use attachments like brushes or nozzles, as these concentrate the heat too much, or to hold the dryer any closer than six inches from the hair. Heated hair rollers or curling tongs also tend to damage the hair, so use these for special occasions only. Lemon juice combed through the hair after rinsing acts as a natural setting lotion.

In case of dry hair, a conditioner used after shampooing will put some life and lustre into the hair. An occasional oil treatment also helps improve dry hair. A warmed vegetable oil should be applied. It should be massaged in well, and the head should be wrapped in a towel which has been wrung out in hot water. This should be left on for at least a quarter of an hour before shampooing. Lemon juice in the final rinse will help to remove any last traces of oil.

An egg yolk is a gentle cleanser which especially suits dry hair. One or two egg yolks should be mixed with a little warm water. The water should not be too hot. This mixture should be applied to the hair. Wrap a towel round the head and leave the mixture on for several minutes before rinsing thoroughly. There is no need to apply any other shampoo.

Home Remedies

Certain herbs and natural substances have been found useful in giving shine and lustre to the hair. One such method is to add a few tea leaves to a glass of water and to then heat it. The juice of a lime should be squeezed in the sieved mixture and the mixture should be applied to the hair before shampooing.

The juice of celery leaves *(ajwain ka patta)* helps to grow long and lustrous hair. Two or three handfuls of celery leaves should be boiled in water. It should then be cooled and strained. The juice of lime should be added to it. This mixture should be used to rinse the hair after washing.

Dry peels of lemons and oranges can also be used beneficially to give lustre and shine to the hair. These peels should be used with soap-nut *(reetha)* or *shikakai,* while shampooing the hair. This will maintain soft and silky hair and also remove dandruff from the scalp.

Rinsing the hair with the juice of a lemon or vinegar also gives lustre to the hair. Add lemon-juice or vinegar to half a bucket of water. After washing the hair, rinse it with this water.

Castor oil, being unsaturated, can be used to rejuvenate the hair. It can be used externally by rubbing it into the scalp at bedtime, and the hair should be washed the next morning. Alternatively, the oil may be rubbed into the scalp and a large towel which has been dipped in hot water and wrung out, may be tied around the head for a while. This allows greater penetration of the oil deep into the surface of the scalp.

Colouring

Permanent dyes are harmful to the hair, as they penetrate the hair cortex layer with the aid of hydrogen peroxide, destroy the keratin structure and create porosity. These dyes gradually eat away and destroy the delicate structure of the hair. This is true of semi-permanent dyes also.

Herbs, which are comparatively safe and healthy, have been used for many centuries as colouring agents. The best-known of these is henna *(mehndi)*. Indian women apply it not only to their hands and feet on auspicious occasions, but also use it for colouring hair. Being a natural colouring agent, its use is not restricted to the young but also to the old well past their middle-age.

Henna is completely organic and comes in a powder form with a smell faintly resembling that of hay.

Henna, if used carefully and sensibly, can do more than just colour the hair. Like semi-permanent colour, it coats the hair shaft, but normally does not penetrate it. Because of this coating action, henna gives the hair a little bulk and body and thus it is also useful as a conditioner. It has a drying effect on the scalp and hence it controls an oily condition of the hair. It gives extra shine to the hair when used the first time, provided an egg and lemon juice is added to it. But repeated application will cause a build up that coats the hair and gives an appearance of dullness. For this reason, the application of henna should be restricted to about four times a year.

Protection Against The Sun

The hair is constantly exposed to the environment as very few of us cover our hair. It can be damaged by over-exposure to the sun. The sun dries the hair, makes it dull, causes breakage and frays the ends. Sun-damaged hair is weak and unhealthy. It is therefore

70

essential to protect the hair from the sun by covering it with a scarf or hat or by using an umbrella.

CHAPTER 11

HAIR DISORDERS
AND THEIR NATURAL TREATMENT

The hair, like the skin, is a barometer to the state of general health. Sickness, deficiencies and mental tension have an adverse effect on the health of the hair and lead to hair disorders. The more important of these disorders are dandruff, loss of hair and premature greying. These disorders and the natural remedies for their treatment are discussed in this chapter.

1. Dandruff

Dandruff refers to the flaking of the scalp which falls like snow flakes and settles on one's brows, shoulders and clothes. It is the greatest enemy of healthy hair. It assumes an unpleasant, irritating condition associated with bacteria in the case of excessive formation of scales on the scalp. These scales are formed from the horny layer of the skin.

The scaliness increases whenever the hair is brushed or rubbed. It may also appear as lumps or crusts on the scalp. Often there is itching as well, and the scalp may become red from scratching.

The main causes of dandruff are impairment of general health, toxic condition of the system brought on mainly by wrong feeding, constipation and lowered vitality due to infectious diseases.

Other factors contributing to dandruff are emotional

tension, harsh shampoos, exposure to cold and general exhaustion.

Natural Remedies

Numerous medicated shampoos are available in the market for the treatment of dandruff. Most of these, however, in the process of curing the disorder, cause irreparable damage to hair roots because of the synthetic ingredients contained in them. The treatment of dandruff has to be largely constitutional if a permanent cure is desired.

The foremost consideration in the treatment of this disorder is to keep the hair and scalp clean so as to minimise the accumulation of dead cells. The hair should be brushed daily to improve the circulation and remove any flakiness. The scalp should also be thoroughly massaged every day, using one's fingertips and working systematically over the head. The procedure for massaging the scalp has been explained in the previous chapter.

Several home remedies have been found useful for treating dandruff. The use of fenugreek *(methi)* seeds is one such remedy. Two tablespoons of these seeds should be soaked overnight in water. The softened seeds should be ground into a fine paste in the morning and applied all over the scalp. It should be left on for half an hour, and the hair should then be washed thoroughly with soap-nut *(reetha)* solution or shikakai.

The use of a teaspoon of fresh lime juice for the last rinse, while washing the hair, is equally beneficial. This not only leaves the hair glowing but also removes stickiness and prevents dandruff. Washing the hair twice a week with green gram *(mung)* powder mixed in curd is another useful prescription.

Dandruff can be removed by massaging one's hair for half an hour with curd which has been kept in the open for three days, or with a few drops of lime juice mixed with *amla* juice every night before going to bed. Another measure which helps to counteract dandruff is to dilute cider vinegar with an equal quantity of water and dab this on to the hair with cotton wool in between shampooing. Cider vinegar added to the final rinse after shampooing also helps to disperse dandruff.

Dietary Consideration

Diet plays an important role in the treatment of dandruff. To begin with, the patient should resort to an all-fruit diet for about five days. In this regimen, there should be three meals a day, consisting of fresh, juicy fruits, such as apples, pears, grapes, grapefruit, pineapple and peaches. Bananas and dried, stewed or tinned fruits should not be taken. During this period, a warm water enema should be taken daily to cleanse the bowels and all other measures adopted to eradicate constipation.

After the all-fruit diet, the patient can gradually adopt a well-balanced diet. Emphasis should be on raw foods, especially fresh fruits and vegetables, sprouted seeds, raw nuts and whole grain cereals, particularly millet and brown rice. Further short periods on the all-fruit diet for three days or so may be necessary at a monthly interval, till the skin's condition improves.

Strict attention to diet is essential for recovery. Starchy, protein and fatty foods should be restricted. Meats, sugar, strong tea or coffee, condiments, pickles and refined and processed foods should be avoided, as also soft drinks, candies, ice-cream and all products made with sugar and white flour.

Exposure of the head to the rays of the sun is also a useful measure in the treatment of dandruff. Simultaneously, an attempt should be made to keep the body in good health. This also helps clear dandruff.

2. Loss Of Hair

Loss of hair at a very early age has become a common disorder these days. It causes a great deal of concern to the affected persons, esp cially Indian women who regard thick long hair as a sign of beauty.

The most important cause of loss of hair is inadequate nutrition. Even a partial lack of almost any nutrient may cause hair to fall. Persons lacking vitamin B6 lose their hair and those deficient in folic acid become completely bald. But the hair grows normally after the liberal intake of these vitamins.

Another important cause for the falling of hair is stress, such as worry, anxiety and sudden shock. Stress leads to severe tension in the skin of the scalp. This adversely affects the supply of essential nutrition required for the healthy growth of hair. General debility, caused by severe or long-standing illnesses like typhoid, syphilis, chronic cold, influenza and anaemia, also gives rise to this hair disorder. It makes the roots of the hair weak, resulting in the falling of hair. An unclean condition of the scalp can also cause the loss of hair. It weakens the hair roots by blocking the pores with the collected dirt. Heredity is another predisposing factor which may cause hair to fall.

Treatment

The healthy condition of the hair depends, to a very large extent, on the intake of sufficient amounts of essential nutrients in the daily diet. Hair is made of protein and adequate protein is necessary for luxuriant hair. Women require 60 grams, men 80 to 90 and adolescent boys and girls 80 to 100 grams of protein. Protein is supplied by milk, buttermilk, yoghurt, soyabean, eggs, cheese, meat and fish. A lack of vitamin A may cause the hair to be coarse and ugly. A deficiency of some of the B vitamins, of iron, copper and iodine may cause hair disorders like falling of hair and premature greying of hair.

Women are generally deficient in iodine and vitamin B1, either of which slow down circulation to the scalp to such an extent that hair may fall out and new hair grows in very slowly. Women who keep their diets adequate in iodine, the B vitamins and iron have better growth of hair.

Lack of inositol causes loss of hair. A person having trouble with his or her hair should eat foods rich in inositol such as yeast, liver and molasses.

Natural Remedies.

Several natural remedies have been found useful in the prevention and treatment of loss of hair. The most effective among these remedies is a vigorous rubbing of the scalp with fingertips after washing the hair with cold water. The scalp should be rubbed vigorously till it starts to tingle with the heat. It will activate the sebaceous glands and energise the circulation of blood in the affected area, making the hair growth healthy.

The oil from the Indian gooseberry *(amla)*, prepared by boiling dry pieces of *amla* in coconut oil, is considered a valuable hair tonic for enriching hair growth. A mixture of equal quantities of fresh *amla* juice, and lime juice used as a shampoo stimulates hair growth and prevents hair loss.

Lettuce *(salad-ka-patta)* is useful in preventing hair loss through deficiencies. A mixture of lettuce and spinach juice is said to help the growth of hair if drunk to the extent of half-a-litre a day. The juice of alfalfa (lucerne) in combination with these juices is rich in elements which are particularly useful for the growth of hair. While preparing alfalfa juice, fresh leaves of the plant should be used.

Daily application of refined coconut oil, mixed with lime water and lime juice on the hair, prevents loss of hair and lengthens it. Application of the juice of green coriander leaves on the head is also considered beneficial.

Mustard oil, boiled with henna *(mehndi)* leaves, is

78

useful for the healthy growth of hair. About 250 grams of mustard oil should be boiled in a tin basin. A little quantity of henna leaves should be gradually put in this oil till about 60 grams of these leaves are thus burnt in the oil. The oil should then be filtered through a cloth and stored well in a bottle. Regular massage of the head with this oil will produce abundant hair.

Another effective remedy for loss of hair is the application of coconut milk all over the scalp and massaging it into the hair roots. It will nourish the hair and promote hair growth. Coconut milk is prepared by grinding coconut shavings and squeezing it well.

Washing the hair with a paste of cooked black gram *(urad dal)* and fenugreek *(methi)* leaves lengthens the hair. A fine paste made from pigeon pea or red gram *(arhar dal)* can also be applied regularly with beneficial results on bald patches. Regular use of castor oil as a hair oil helps the luxuriant growth of the hair.

Certain remedies have also been found useful in case of patchy loss of hair. The seeds of lime and black pepper seeds, ground to a fine paste, is a valuable remedy. This paste, applied on the patches, has a mildly irritant action. This increases blood circulation to the affected areas and stimulates hair growth. The paste should be applied twice a day for a few weeks.

Another useful remedy for the patchy loss of hair is the paste of liquorice *(mulethi)* made by grinding the pieces in milk with a pinch of saffron. This paste should be applied over the bald patches before going to bed at night.

3. Premature Greying Of Hair.

The hair has a tendency to lose its natural colour with advancing age. It is therefore natural for the hair to turn grey with age. But premature greying is a morbid condition and it makes even the young look older.

Faulty diet and worries are the two primary causes of premature greying of hair. It is mainly due to the lack of some of the B vitamins, of iron, copper and iodine in the daily diet that leads to his hair disorder at a young age. Worries produce an extraordinary tension in the skin of the scalp which interferes with the supply of vital nutrition necessary for the health of hair. Similarly, anxieties, fear, jealousy and failures have adverse effects on the hair. They dry out the scalpular marrow, the vital sap at the root of the hair.

Other causes for premature greying of hair are the unclean condition of the scalp which weakens the roots of the hair as the pores are blocked by the collected dirt; washing the hair with hot water and drying it with electric dryers which emit a blast of hot air; use of hairdyes when the hair has just started greying; diseases like chronic cold, sinusitis, anaemia, chronic constipation; and the use of factory-made hair oils, which are generally cleaned with acids which have a tendency to remain in the oil. Heredity is yet another predisposing factor which gives rise to this ailment.

Natural Remedies

Certain home remedies have been found useful in the prevention and treatment of premature greying of the hair. The foremost among these is the use of the Indian gooseberry *(amla)* which is a valuable hair tonic for enriching hair growth and hair pigmentation. The fruit, cut into pieces, should be dried, preferably in the shade. These pieces should be boiled in coconut oil till the solid matter becomes like charred dust. This darkish oil is very useful in preventing greying.

The water in which dried *amla* pieces are soaked overnight is also nourishing for the hair. This water should be used as the last rinse while washing the hair. Massaging the scalp with a teaspoon of *amla* juice, mixed with a teaspoon of almond oil or a few drops of lime juice, every night, has proved beneficial in the prevention and treatment of premature greying of hair.

Amaranth *(chaulai-ka-saag)* is useful in hair disorders. Application of the fresh juice of the leaves of this vegetable helps the hair to retain its black colour and prevents premature greying. It also helps the growth of hair and keeps it soft.

Liberal intake of curry leaves is considered benefical in preventing premature greying of hair. These leaves give vitality and strength to hair roots. New hair roots that grow are healthier with normal pigment. The leaves can be used in the form of a chutney or may be squeezed in buttermilk. When the leaves are boiled in coconut oil, the oil forms an excellent hair tonic to stimulate hair growth and bring back hair pigmentation.

Ribbed gourd *(torai)* boiled in coconut oil is another effective remedy for premature greying of hair. Pieces of this vegetable should be dried in the shade. These dried pieces should be soaked in coconut oil and kept aside for three or four days. The oil should then be boiled till the mass is reduced to a blackened residue. This oil should be massaged into the scalp. It will help enrich the hair roots and restore pigment to the hair.

Hair Dye

A paste of henna leaves, boiled in coconut oil to get a darkish oil, can be used as a hair dye to blacken grey hair. The paste itself can be applied to the hair and washed away after a few hours. Washing the hair with concentrated tea extract twice a week is also considered useful in colouring grey hair to brown or black.

Walnut shells also make a harmless hair dye, which progressively adds colour to the hair. Before the nuts are ripe, the green outer shells should be crushed in a mortar and covered with water. A pinch of salt should be added. This should be allowed to stay for three days. Then, three cups of boiling water should be added and simmered for five hours, making sure to replace the evaporated water. The dark liquid should be extracted by twisting the shells in a cloth. The separated liquid should be replaced in a pot again and reduced to a quarter of its volume. A little alum and glycerine should be added to soften the hair. At first, it will produce a somewhat yellowish effect, but it will finally give the hair a good deep black colour.

Dietary Consideration

Diet is of utmost importance in the prevention and

treatment of premature greying of hair, and persons suffering from this disorder should take a diet rich in all essential nutrients. The vitamins considered useful in premature greying of hair are pantothenic acid, para-aminobenzoic acid or paba and inositol. To obtain satisfactory results, all three of these vitamins, belonging to the B group, should be supplied at one time, preferably in a form which gives all B vitamins, such as yeast and liver. The three anti-grey hair vitamins can also be produced in the intestinal tract by bacteria. Thus drinking a sufficient quantity of yoghurt daily and having a tablespoon of yeast before each meal will be an excellent remedy for the prevention and treatment of premature greying of hair.

Devitalised foods like white flour, refined sugar, and all products made from them, soft drinks, pastries, jams and jellies should be avoided. These foods, besides causing premature grey hair, take away energy, bring about wrinkles, unattractive skin, and premature old age.

CHAPTER 12

CARING FOR HANDS AND FEET

Beautiful hands are an essential complement to a woman's beauty. With proper care, almost any pair of hands can look beautful. The state of one's hands cannot be kept hidden from view, however much one may try to do so. As with most things, preventing trouble is considerably easier than curing it.

The hands and fingers are one of the busiest parts of the body. They are exposed to all kinds of weather conditions. They also constantly come in contact with water which contains such powerful chemical solutions as washing powder, bleach and washing-up liquids. The hands are therefore one of the first parts of the body to show signs of neglect and ageing. The guidelines for keeping them in proper shape are discussed herein.

Protection

The most important factor for proper care of hands is that they should be properly dried with a towel after every contact with water. The longer the water remains on the skin the more dehydrating it is. It is essential to protect them in such a way that they do not come into direct contact with a constant barrage of chemicals. A pair of rubber gloves should be worn for all household chores like washing and cleaning. One may feel uncomfortable, but will get used to it if a pair of fine rubber gloves is chosen. Cotton gloves can be worn for jobs where the hands do not come in contact with water.

Cleansing

Each night the hands should be washed with a mild soap and scrubbed thoroughly with a face brush. In case of hard skin, it should be whizzed over with a pumice stone. If the fingers are stained due to vegetables or nicotine, they should be rubbed with lime. This will help bleach the stain. They should then be rinsed well and dried thoroughly.

The hands should be treated once or twice a week to a massage with a really rich cream. This should be preceded by soaking them in warm oil, preferably olive or almond, for five to 30 minutes.

This is a good treatment for dry hands and nails.

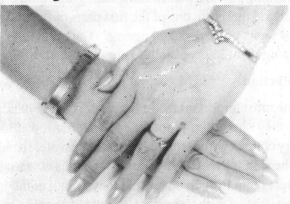

Beautiful hands are an essential complement to a woman's beauty.

CARING FOR HANDS AND FEET

Care For Finger Nails

Like the hair, nails are composed of keratin which is formed mainly from protein and calcium. Therefore a diet rich in these two nutrients is an essential part of healthy nails. Nails that are in poor condition are indicative of poor general health.

Like the hands, the fingers nails are constantly subjected to abuse. So any hand care programe should incorporate the nails. They will benefit from regular applications of a rich moisturizer such as a night cream.

An orange stick tipped with cotton wool should be used to clean beneath the nails. An orange stick should be used to gently shape the cuticles, to avoid breaking or tearing of the skin. The best time to shape the cuticles is after the hands have been in water, as it softens the skin and makes the cuticles ready for shaping. Alternatively, the fingers can be soaked in a little vegetable oil, or in warm water and herbal shampoo for a few minutes.

Drinking cider vinegar each day is believed to help strengthen the nails, as well as being good for general health. A tablespoon of the vinegar should be taken in a glass of water three times a day before meals.

A useful remedy for keeping the hands young and beautiful is to dip them upto the wrist, in a bowl of milk. Then blot and apply three tablespoons of lanolin mixed with one tablespoon of sesame oil *(til)* on the hands and wrists. This should be done once a week.

Exercising the hands helps to make them flexible and

improves circulation. The following exercises may be done, repeating them six to ten times:

1. Clench your fists tightly for a second. Then throw open the fingers as wide as possible.

2. Put your hands out in front of you, palm down. Press the fingers tightly against each other and then thrust them apart as wide as possible.

3. Allow the hands to be limp and relaxed. Then rotate them from the wrists in circles, first clockwise and then anti-clockwise.

If the hands are tired, soak them for a few minutes in warm water, to which about two or three tablespoons of salt have been added. This helps to soothe them. Another treatment which stimulates circulation is to soak the hands alternatively in hot and cold water. This also soothes the nerve endings.

Care For Feet

One should not forget about looking after the feet because they are hidden. They need regular care not only to make them look good but also to avoid such crippling conditions like corns and callouses, which can lead to painful feet. Besides, the strain of tired and aching feet will adversely affect even the most beautiful face. It will also cause a loss of balance while walking and promote tension and irritability.

Ill-fitting shoes are the most likely cause of foot problems. Shoes should therefore be always chosen for comfort. They should support the arch of the foot well and should allow ample room for the toes. Shoes with high heels and pointed toes should never be worn as these prove harmful.

Like the hands, the feet should be kept in good shape with a few simple exercises. A useful exercise for the feet is to arch the ankles, bend the toes and flex the whole foot first thing in the morning. Walking is one of the best exercises for the feet. Feet that are sore and swollen after a long day, should be relaxed by placing them higher than the head and gently massaging them. In case of cold feet a massage with olive oil will help greatly. An ancient remedy for tired feet is to soak them alternately in hot and cold water, finishing with the cold water. Soaking the feet in warm water, to which Epsom salts or special foot salts have been added, can be very soothing, but the feet should be rubbed over afterwards with eau-de-cologne to counteract any softening effect.

The toe nails should be given as much attention as the nails of the hands. An orange stick tipped with cotton wool should be used to clean around the nails. Particular attention should be paid to the sides of the nails where dirt tends to collect. Thereafter, a generous amount of moisturizing body lotion should be rubbed all over the feet.

To keep the feet smelling fresh, especially in hot weather, a deodorizing talcum powder should be applied each morning after washing. Socks, if used, should be washed daily.

The knees also need to be looked after. The should be made wet and rubbed thoroughly with two tablespoons of powdered groundnut mixed with a tablespoon of salt. After a few minutes, they should be rinsed and a film of sesame oil mixed with a few drops of vinegar should be applied. Regular massage in this manner will keep them in good condition.

CHAPTER 13

THE NATURAL WAY TO SLIMMING

Obesity and beauty do not go together. It is difficult to look beautiful with bulges in the wrong places. Excess weight affects the face and figure. It also shakes one's self confidence. Pride in one's appearance plays an important part in being beautiful.

Obesity is also a serious health hazard as the extra fat puts a strain on the heart, kidneys and liver, as well as on the large weight-bearing joints such as the hips, knees and ankles. This ultimately shortens the life span. It has been rightly said, 'the longer the belt, the shorter the life'. Overweight persons are susceptible to several diseases like coronary thrombosis, heart failure, high blood pressure, diabetes, arthritis, gout, liver and gall-bladder disorders. Trimming your figure is, therefore, necessary for the sake of both goods looks and health.

The chief cause of obesity, most often, is overeating that is, the intake of calories beyond the body's energy requirement. Some persons are in the habit of eating much, while others may be in the habit of consuming high calorie foods. These persons gain weight continuously as they fail to adjust their appetite to reduced energy requirements. There has, in recent times, been an increasing awareness of the psychological aspects of obesity. Persons who are generally unhappy, lonely or unloved and those who are discontented with their families, or social or financial standing, usually take solace in over-eating.

Obesity is sometimes also the result of disturbances of the thyroid or pituitary gland. But glandular disorders account for only about two per cent of the total incidence of obesity. In such persons the metabolism rate is low and they keep gaining weight unless they take a low calorie diet.

Natural Remedies

Many diets are prescribed for the overweight to enable them to reduce. Some of these diets are so severe and extreme that they are likely to be more detrimental to health than being overweight. Crash diets which severely restrict food intake or exclude all but one or two items are injurious to health, irrespective of the seriousness of the problem of obesity. Not only is the health likely to suffer but the person adhering to such a diet is likely to put on many of those lost kilos back again after resumption of normal eating habits.

Another risk with most diets is that in cutting down on the amount of food, they drastically reduce the intake of vital nutrients and this may lead to tiredness and irritability. The only sensible way to lose weight and to maintain that weight loss is to follow a carefully planned course of dietetic treatment, in conjunction with suitable exercise and other measures for promoting good health. The chief consideration in this treatment should be the balanced selection of foods which provide the maximum essential nutrients with the least number of calories.

To begin with, the patient should undertake a juice fast for seven to ten days. Juices of lemon, grapefruit, orange, pineapple cabbage and carrots may be taken during this period. A longer juice fast upto 40 days can also be undertaken but only under expert guidance and supervision. Alternatively, short juice fasts should be repeated at regular intervals of two months or so till the desired reduction in weight is achieved.

After the juice fast, the patient should spend the next four or five days on an all-fruit diet, taking three meals of fresh juicy fruits such as orange, grapefruit, pineapple and papaya. Thereafter, he may gradually start on a low calorie, well balanced diet of whole grains, vegetables and fruits, with emphasis on raw fruits, vegetables and fresh juices.

The foods which should be drastically curtailed or altogether avoided are high-fat foods such as butter, cheese, chocolate, cream, ice-cream, fatty meats, fried foods and gravies; foods high in carbohydrates like bread, candy, cakes, cookies, cereal products, legumes, potatoes, honey, sugar, syrup and rich puddings; beverages such as aerated drinks and alcohol.

Tea and coffee should be eliminated completely. If this is not possible, they should be restricted to one or two cups a day. Herbal teas can be taken as they do not contain calories provided no sweetener is added. Lemon juice also acts as a diuretic and can be taken for this purpose first thing in the morning with hot water. Having something to drink half-an-hour before a meal also helps to take the edge off your appetite. Skimmed milk should be used in place of whole milk as this is much lower in calorie. If some snack needs to be eaten between meals, raw fruits or vegetables are preferable to biscuits and cakes. All foods should be cooked carefully to retain maximum nutrient content, without increasing the calories. This means eating raw or steamed vegetables. Nutritious but high calorie foods, such as nuts, hard cheese, commercial fruits, yoghurt and avocado pears, should be avoided. Lots of salad should be included in the diet as they are low in calories and a good source of vitamins and minerals.

Fletcherism

One sure method of reducing weight is by practising what is known as 'Fletcherism'. It was discovered in 1898 by Horace Fletcher of the U.S.A. Fletcher, at 40, considered himself an old man. He was 25 kilos overweight, contracted flu every six months and constantly complained of indigestion and exhaustion. After deep study, he discovered the rules for 'Fletcherism' which are as follows:

1. Chew your food to a pulp or milky liquid until it practically swallows itself.

2. Never eat until hungry.

3. Enjoy every bite or morsel, savouring the flavour until it is swallowed.

4. Do not eat when tired, angry, worried and at meal times refuse to think or talk about unpleasant subjects.

Horace Fletcher followed these rules for five months. As a result, he lost more than 27 kilos and felt better than he had for 20 years. A weight-reducing programme built on Fletcherism works wonders and is worth a trial.

Along with dietetic treatment, the patient should adopt all other natural methods of reducing weight. Exercise is an important part of the weight reduction plan. It helps to use calories stored in body fat and relieves tension, besides toning up the muscles of the body. Walking is the best exercise to begin with and may be followed by running, swimming, rowing and other outdoor sports.

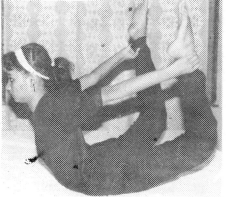

Yogic asanas like dhanurasana break up fatty deposits and help in losing weight.

Certain yogic *asanas* are highly beneficial. Not only do they break up or re-distribute fatty deposits and help slimming, but they also strenghten the flabby areas. These *asanas* include *shalabhasana, dhanurasana, chakrasana, vajrasana, yogamudra* and *trikonasana.*

These *asanas* work on the glands, improve circulation, strengthen many weak areas and induce deep breathing which helps to melt off excess fat gradually. The methods for practising these asanas have been given in Chapter 15, 'Yoga For Youthful Looks'.

Above all, the obese person should make every effort to avoid negative emotions such as anxiety, fear, hostility and insecurity and develop a positive outlook towards life.

CHAPTER 14

EXERCISE FOR BEAUTY

Gone are the days when physical exercise was considered to be for those who wished to lose weight. There is now growing awareness that physical fitness and exercise play a vital role for the attainment and maintenance of good health, good looks and youthfulness. It it also a wonderful way to have a good figure.

This is based on the realisation that negative influences adversely affect the health and beauty of a person and lead to degeneration of the human body. Factors like environmental pollution, exposure to chemicals and drugs, synthetic foods, sedentary life style and mental stress undermine health and good loods and increase the incidence of degenerative diseases, thereby hastening the ageing process.

Exercise is a key factor in the search for a youthful appearance. It relieves tension, anxiety and stress which greatly contribute to premature wrinkling. There is a close relationship between exercise and healthy skin.

Exercise enables a person to attain a state of well-being which protects the body from degeneration. It is a level of good health that helps to counteract the ageing changes in the body and also allows both body and mind to function efficiently.

Benefits
The body benefits from exercise in various ways. The

different systems of the body get a boost and this results in their better functioning, increased strength, stamina and energy. It improves circulation of the blood, facilitates better transportation of oxygen and nutrients to all parts of the body, right up to the skin. This enables the skin to eliminate the waste in a more efficient way, thereby preserving it from ageing changes.

The improved circulation and optimum oxygenation helps to counteract may circulatory problems associated with age. Exercise improves the tone and elasticity of muscles and joints. This enables the body to look and feel young and gives the figure good proportions.

Regular exercise also enables the body to achieve poise, grace and a good posture which are essential factors for good looks and youthful appearance. It thus helps to delay ageing. Regular exercise programmes have shown remarkable improvement in health and appearance.

Methods Of Exercise

Several systems of exercise have been developed over the years, the most popular among them being the Swedish system and yoga *asanas*, the latter having been practised from ancient times. Whichever system one chooses to adopt, the exercises should be performed systematically, regularly and under proper guidance.

To be really useful, exercise should be taken in such a manner as to bring into action all the muscles of the body in a natural way. Walking is one such exercise. It is the most efficient exercise for improving overall fitness. It uses more muscles in a continuous, uniform action than most other forms of exercise and it remains accessible to everyone throughout life. A regular walking programme can help one lose weight, give more energy and tone flabby muscles. It can help prevent heart disease, alleviate mental depression and ease some of the pain of arthritis as well as reverse some of the physical aspects of ageing. This form of exercise is, however, so gentle in character that one must walk several kilometres in a brisk manner to constitute a fair amount of exercise. Other forms of good exercise are swimming, cycling, horseriding, tennis, etc.

Precautions.

Vigorous exercise of any kind should not be taken for an hour-and-a-half after eating, nor immediately before meals. Weak patients and those suffering from serious diseases like cancer, heart trouble, tuberculosis and asthma should not undertake vigorous exercise except under the supervision of a competent physician.

If exercising makes you tired, stop immediately. The purpose of exercise should be to make you feel refreshed and relaxed and not tired.

The most important rule of the fitness plan is to start with very light exercise and to increase the effort in gradual and easy stages. The sense of well-being will begin almost immediately. One can start off with a brisk walk for 15 to 20 minutes. A comfortable sense of tiredness should be the aim. It is valuable and possibly harmful to become exhausted or seriously short of breath. Perhaps, one should aim at activities which need about two-third of one's maximum ability. One way to assess is to count your own pulse rate.

Counting the pulse rate is quite easy. Feel the pulse on your left wrist with the middle three fingers of your right hand. Press just firmly enough to feel the beat easily. Now count the number of beats in 15 seconds, with the help of a watch with a second hand, and calculate your rate by multiplying by four. At rest your heart beats 70 to 80 times a minute. This rate increases during exercise. Really vigorous exercise can produce rates as high as 200 beats or more per minute. A reasonable aim is to exercise at about two-thirds of your maximum capacity. It follows that the heart rate should be about 130 per minute during and just after exercise. Always avoid over-exertion and never allow your pulse to go above 190 minus your age per minute.

CHAPTER 15

YOGA FOR YOUTHFUL LOOKS

The term 'yoga' is derived from the Sanskrit root 'yug' which means 'to join'. It signifies union between the individual soul *(jivatma)* and the Universal Soul *(Parmatma)*. It is an ancient system of discipline practised in India. Many references to yoga have been made in the Upanishads. It was, however, Maharishi Patanjali who gave a systematic treatment to the traditional yogic teachings around the first century B.C.

Yoga aims at the entire well-being of man. Basically, human evolution takes place on three different planes, namely physical, mental and spiritual. Yoga is a means of attaining perfect health by maintaining harmony and achieving optimum functioning on all three levels through complete self-control.

The practice of yoga *asanas* leads to a well-balanced personality. It improves circulation and energises and stimulates major endocrine glands of the body. Yogic exercises promote inner health and harmony, and their regular practice helps prevent and cure many common ailments. They also help eliminate tensions, be they physical, mental and emotional. They improve suppleness, grace and posture and keep the spine flexible. They are said to beautify the face and figure and delay old age.

All yogic exercises should be performed on a clean mat, carpet or blanket covered with a cotton sheet.

Clothing should be light and loose-fitting to allow free movement of the limbs. The mind should be kept off all disturbances and tensions. Regularity and punctuality in practising yogic exercises is essential.

Yoga *asanas* should be practised only after mastering the techniques with the help of a competent teacher. *Asanas* should always be practised on an empty stomach, and at a leisurely slow-motion pace, maintaining poise and balance.

Certain yogic *asanas* which are highly beneficial for the maintenance of good health and for a youthful appearance are described herein:

1. *Shavasana* **(Dead body pose)** : Lie flat on your back, feet comfortably apart, arms and hands extended about six inches from the body, palms upwards and

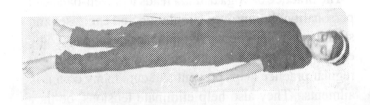

Shavasana

fingers half-folded. Close your eyes. Begin by consciously and gradually relaxing every part and each muscle of the body - feet, legs, calves, knees, thighs, abdomen, hips, back, hands, arms, chest, shoulders, neck, head and face. Relax completely feeling as if your whole body is lifeless. Now concentrate on breathing rhythmically, as slowly and effortlessly as possible. This creates a state of complete relaxation. Remain motionless in this position, relinquishing all responsibilities and worries for 10 to 15 minutes. Discontinue the exercise when your legs grow numb. This *asana* relaxes the mind and soothes the nervous system. It should be performed at the beginning and at the end of the daily round of yogic *asanas*.

2. *Yogamudra* : Sit erect in *padmasana* (lotus posture). Fold your hands behind your back, holding your left wrist with the right hand. Take a deep breath. While

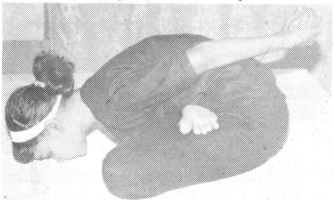

Yogamudra

exhaling, bend forward slowly keeping your hands on your back. Bring your face downwards until your nose and forehead touch the floor. While inhaling, slowly rise back to the upright position. The practise of this *asana* tones the nervous system, builds up powerful abdomi-

103

nal muscles and strengthens the pelvic organs. It helps pep up digestion, boosts the appetite and removes constipation.

3. *Vajrasana* (Pelvic pose) : Sit erect and stretch out your legs. Fold your legs back, placing feet on the sides of the buttocks with the soles facing back and upwards.

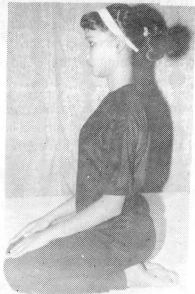

Vajrasana

Rest your buttocks on the floor between your heels. The toes of both feet should touch. Now, place your hands on your knees and keep the spine, neck and head straight. This *asana* can be performed even after meals. It improves digestion and is beneficial in case of stiffness of the legs. It strengthens the hips, thighs, knees, calves, ankles and toes.

4. *Sarvangasana* **(Shoulder stand pose)** : In San-skrit, *'sarva'* means whole and *'anga'* means limb. Almost all parts of the body are involved in and benefit from this *asana.* Lie flat on your back with your arms by the side, palms turned down. Bring your legs up slowly to a 90° angle and then raise the rest of the body by pushing the legs up and resting their weight on the arms. Fix your chin in the jugular notch, and use your

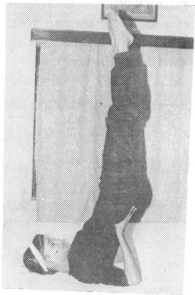

Sarvangasana

arms and hands to support the body at the hip region. The weight of the body should rest on your head, back and shoulders, your arms being used merely for balance. The trunk and legs should be in a straight line. The body, legs, hips and trunk should be kept as vertical as possible. Focus your eyes on your big toes. Press your chin against your chest. Hold the pose for one to three minutes. Return to the starting position slowly reversing the procedure.

Sarvangasana stimulates the thyroid and para-thyroid glands, influences the brain and strengthens the mind.

5. *Halasana* (Plough pose) : Lie flat on your back with legs and feet together, arms by your side with fists closed near your thigh, keeping your legs straight; slowly raise them to angles of 30°, 60° and 90°, pausing slightly at each point. Gradually, raise your legs above

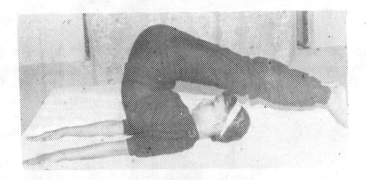

Halasana

your head without bending your knees and then move them behind until they touch the floor. Stretch your legs as far as possible so that your chin presses tightly against the chest while your arms remain on the floor as in the original position. Hold the pose from between 10 seconds to three minutes, breathing normally. To return to the starting position, slowly reverse the procedure. This *asana* relieves tension in the back, neck and legs.

6. *Bhujangasana* **(Cobra pose)** : Lie on your stomach with your legs straight and feet together, toes pointing backwards. Rest your forehead and nose on the ground. Place your palms below the shoulders and your arms by the side of the chest. Inhale and slowly

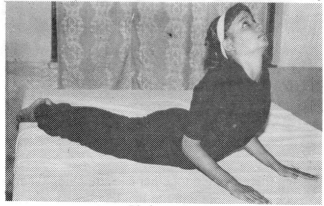

Bhujangasana

raise your head, neck, chest and upper abdomen from the navel up. Bend your spine back and arch your back as far as you can, looking upwards. Maintain this position and hold your breath for a few seconds. Exhale, and slowly return to the original position. This *asana* removes weakness of the abdomen and tones up the reproductive system in women. It exercises the vertebrae, back muscles and the spine.

7. *Shalabhasana* **(Locust pose)** : Lie flat on your stomach, with your legs stretched out straight, feet together, chin and nose resting on the ground, looking straight ahead. Move your arms under the body, keeping them straight, fold your hands into fists and place them close to the thighs. Now, raise your legs up

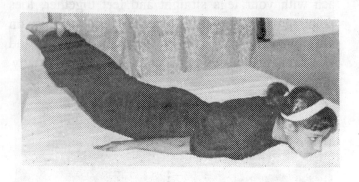

Shalabhasana

keeping them straight together and stretching them as far back as possible without bending your knees and toes. Hold this position for a few seconds and repeat four or five times. This *asana* strengthens the whole body especially the waist, chest, back and neck.

8. *Dhanurasana* (**Bow pose**) : Lie on your stomach with your chin resting on the ground, arms extended alongside the body with the legs straight. Bend your legs back towards the hips, bring them forward and grasp your ankles. Inhale and raise your thighs, chest and head at the same time. Keep your hands straight. The weight of the body should rest mainly on the navel region. Therefore, arch your spine as much as possible. Exhale and return slowly to the starting position, by reversing the procedure. *Dhanurasana* provides good exercise for the arms, shoulders, legs, ankles, back and

neck. It also strengthens the spine.

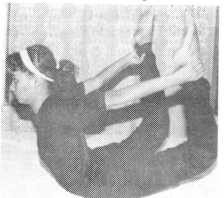

Dhanurasana

9. *Chakrasana* **(Lateral bending pose)** : Stand

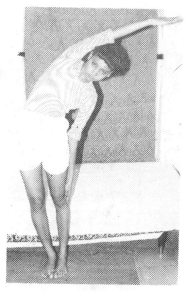

Chakrasana

straight with your feet and toes together and arms by

your sides, palms facing and touching the thighs. Raise one arm laterally above the head with the palm inwards up to shoulder level and palm upwards when the arm rises above the level of your head. Then, bend your trunk and head sideways with the raised arm touching the ear, and sliding the palm of the other hand downwards towards the knee. Keep your knees and elbows straight throughout. Maintain the final pose for a few seconds. Then gradually bring your hand back to the normal position. Repeat the exercise on the other side. This *asana* induces maximum stretching of the lateral muscles of the body, especially the abdomen. It strengthens the knees, arms and shoulders and increases lung capacity.

10. *Trikonasana* (Triangle pose) : Stand erect, with

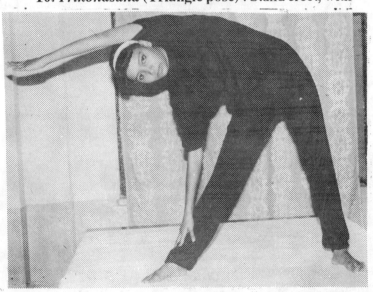

Trikonasana

your legs apart. Stretch your arms up to shoulder level. Bend your trunk forward and twist to the left, looking upwards and keeping your left arm raised at an angle of 90°. Place your right palm on your left foot without bending the knees. Maintain this pose for a few seconds. Then straighten and return to the normal position. Repeat the procedure on the other side. *Trikonasana* is an all-round stretching exercise. It keeps the spinal column flexible and helps reduce the fat on the lateral sides of the body. Besides, it stimulates the adrenal glands and tones the abdominal and pelvic organs.

CHAPTER 16

NATURAL FOODS AS BEAUTY AIDS

There is a wide range of natural foods fruits, vegetables, pulses, nuts, seeds, honey and milk and other products which are of great cosmetic value. They can be benefically used as beauty aids. Some of the important foodstuffs which can be used in this manner are described herein in brief.

FRUITS

Apple *(seb)* : Apple is one of the best fruits to tone a weak and run down condition of the human system. Its regular consumption with milk promotes health and youthfulness and helps build beautiful and bright skin.

Apple is also valuable in keeping teeth in good condition and good teeth are an important part of one's health and appearance. Tooth decay can be prevented by regular consumption of this fruit as it possesses a mouth cleansing property. Taken after meals, it has the same effect as a tooth brush in cleaning the teeth. In addition, the acid contents of the apple promote the flow of saliva in the mouth and exerts influence upon the germs.

Custard Apple *(sitaphal)* : The seeds of the custard apple have detergent properties. Their powder is used to kill lice and prevent dandruff. This powder also serves as a goods hair wash when mixed with Bengal gram flour *(besan)*

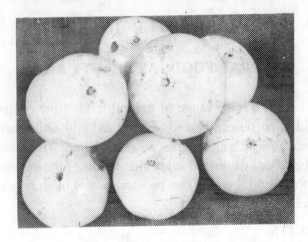

The Indian gooseberry (amla) is an accepted hair tonic

Indian Gooseberry *(amla)* : Indian gooseberry is an accepted hair tonic in traditional recipes for enriching hair growth and hair pigmentation. The fruit, cut into pieces, in dried preferably in the shade. These pieces are boiled in coconut oil till the solid mass becomes like charred dust. This darkish oil is an excellent oil to prevent greying. The water in which dried *amla* pieces are soaked overnight is also nourishing to the hair. This water should be used for the last rinse while washing the hair.

Lemon *(bara nimbu)* : This fruit is regarded as a youth restorative. It helps cleanse blemished skin. The juice should be soaked into the skin, allowing it to remain overnight. Dry or scaly skin can be rubbed with the peel of a lemon. This will restore the skin to softness. Lemon juice can also help brighten the hair. Strained fresh juice of this fruit should be mixed with cool water and used to wash the hair for this purpose. Rough

114

elbows can also be softened by rubbing the area with the cut side of a lemon.

Lime *(nimbu)* : This fruit can also be used as a beauty aid. A fresh lime may be squeezed in a glass of boiled, whole milk. A teaspoon of glycerine may be added to it. It should be left for half an hour and then applied on the face, hands and feet before retiring at night. This will help one to look young and beautiful. The application can also cure pimples, cracked soles and palms, dryness of the face and hands, and protect the face from hot and cold winds and sun-burn. Massaging the scalp with a few drops of lime juice mixed with *amla* juice every night before going to bed, stops the falling of hair, lengthens it and prevents hair from premature greying. It also cures dandruff.

Musk Melon : The vitamin A and C contents of this fruit help rejuvenate internal and external skin tissues. Vitamin C in particular produces collagen, a natural cementing material that holds body cells together, strengthens the walls of the blood vessels in the digestive system and helps in healing the worn out cells and tissues.

Papaya *(papita)* : The juice of the raw papaya, being an irritant, can be applied to swellings to prevent suppuration. It can also be applied beneficially to corns, warts, pimples and horny excrescences of the skin. The juice as a cosmetic, removes freckles and makes the skin smooth and delicate. A paste of the papaya seeds is applied in skin diseases like ringworm.

Peach *(arhu)* : The skin of the peach is useful in improving the complexion. 'A complexion like peaches' is a common expression. The inside of peach peelings should be gently massaged on the face every night for a few minutes. The moisture should not be rubbed off. This will cleanse the skin thoroughly and free the pores. It also has a gentle astringent action and tightens the muscles of the face slightly, thus preventing sagging tissues.

Zizyphus *(ber)* : The paste of the leaves applied over the scalp and hair keeps them clean and prevents scalp diseases. It also lengthens the hair and darkens it.

VEGETABLES

Amaranth *(chaulai-ka-saag)* : This vegetable is useful in hair disorders. Application of the fresh leaf-juice helps the growth of the hair and keeps it soft. It also helps the hair to retain its black colour and prevents premature greying.

The juice applied over the face with a pinch of turmeric powder bleaches the skin, prevents it from dryness and wrinkles, cures pimples and makes one look fresh. This juice, mixed with milk and lime juice, acts as an effective skin tonic to increase and retain the beauty of the skin. It should be delicately massaged over the face and neck for half an hour and washed with lukewarm water every night before going to bed.

Ash Gourd *(safed petha)* : The peel and seeds of the ash gourd, boiled in coconut oil, are useful in hair disorders. They lengthen the hair, prevent dandruff and dryness of the scalp.

Beet *(chukandar)* : A decoction of beets mixed with a little vinegar can be used externally to cleanse scurf and dandruff from the head. For dandruff, the beet water should also be massaged into the scalp every night.

Coriander *(dhania)* : A teaspoon of coriander juice, mixed with a pinch of turmeric powder, is an effective remedy for pimples, blackheads and dry skin. The mixture should be applied to the face after thoroughly washing it, every night before retiring.

Cucumber *(khira)* : Grated cucumber applied over the face, eyes and neck for 15 to 20 minutes has been found effective as a beauty aid and is the best tonic for the skin of the face. Its regular use prevents pimples, blackheads, wrinkles and dryness of the face. Cucumber juice promotes hair growth due to its high silicon and sulphur contents, particularly when mixed with carrot, lettuce and spinach juice.

Curry Leaves *(kurry patta)* : Liberal intake of curry leaves is considered beneficial in preventing the premature greying of hair. These leaves give vitality and strength to hair roots. New hair roots that grow are healthier with normal pigment. The leaves can be used in the form of a chutney or they may be squeezed in buttermilk or *lassi.*

Fenugreek (methi) : A paste of the fresh leaves applied over the scalp regularly, before taking bath, lengthens the hair, preserves its natural colour and keeps it silky soft. A paste of the fresh leaves, applied on the face every night before going to bed and washed off with warm water, prevents pimples, blackheads, dryness of the face, and wrinkles. It improves the complexion and makes one look years younger.

Drumstick *(sanjana)* : Fresh leaf-juice applied with lime juice is useful in the treatment of pimples, black-heads and keeps one's face fresh.

Garlic *(lasoon)* : Garlic has been used successfully for a variety of skin disorders. Pimples disappear without leaving a scar when rubbed with raw garlic several times a day. Even very persistent form of acne, suffered by some adults, has also been healed with garlic. The external use of garlic helps to clear spots on the skin, pimples and boils. The process is further helped by taking the garlic internally to purify the blood stream for a long-term clearance of the skin. A regular course of three garlic capsules per day should help to clear minor skin infections quickly. Garlic rubbed over ringworm, gives relief.

Lettuce *(salad-ka-patta)* : This salad vegetable is useful in preventing hair loss through deficiencies. A mixture of lettuce and spinach juice is said to help the growth of hair if drunk to the extent of half a litre a day.

Mint *(pudina)* : Application of fresh mint juice over the face every night cures pimples and prevents dryness of the skin. The juice is also applied over insect stings, eczema, scabies and contact dermatitis.

Potato *(alu)* : The juice of raw potatoes has also

proved very valuable in clearing skin blemishes. This cleansing results from the high content of potassium, sulphur, phosphorus and chlorine in the potato. These elements are, however, of value only when the potato is raw as in this state they are composed of live organic atoms. In the cooked state, they are converted into inorganic atoms and are of little value cosmetically.

The juicy pulp of the shredded raw potatoes can also be applied as a poultice in clearing the ageing appearance of the skin. Before going to bed, it may be rubbed on the face and other portions of the body, that have wrinkles. It will help 'melt' the wrinkles, banish age spots and clear the skin. The enzymes in raw potato pulp, combined with the vitamin C and the natural starch, help create a skin food that nourishes the starved cellular tissues of the skin. Furthermore, the alkaline juices of the potato promotes an antiseptic action that gives a glowing look of youth. Much of the decaying skin is sloughed off by the acidic portion of the pulp.

Tomato *(tamatar)* : Tomato as an external application can be used as a cosmetic. Its pulp should be applied liberally on the face and left there for an hour and then washed off with warm water. Repeated daily, it will give one a good complexion and remove ugly-looking pimples in a short time.

PULSES

Bengal Gram *(channa)* : The flour of the unroasted Bengal gram *(besan)* is a very effective cleansing agent and its regular use, as a cosmetic, bleaches the skin. In allergic skin diseases like eczema, contact dermatitis and scabies, washing with this flour will bring about good results. This flour is also useful where pimples are concerned. The flour should be mixed with curd to make a paste. This paste should be applied to the face and washed off after sometime. Washing the hair with Bengal gram flour keeps it clean, soft and free from hair diseases.

Black Gram *(urad dal)* : Washing the hair with a paste of cooked black gram *dal* and fenugreek leaves lengthens the hair, keeps it black and cures dandruff.

Green Gram *(mung)* : The flour of the green gram is an excellent detergent and can be used as a substitute for soap. It removes the dirt and does not cause any skin irritation. Its application over the face bleaches the skin and gives one a good complexion. Black gram flour, mixed with green gram paste, when used for washing the hair, lengthens it and prevents dandruff.

Lentil *(masur)* : The flour of lentil mixed with milk cream can be applied with beneficial results as a bleaching cosmetic. It whitens the complexion and prevents wrinkles on the face.

NUTS

Almond *(badam)* : The paste of almonds with milk cream and fresh rose buds paste applied daily over the face is a very effective beauty aid. It softens and bleaches the skin and nourishes it with the choicest skin-food. Its regular application prevents early appearance of wrinkles, blackheads, dryness of the skin, pimples

120

and keeps the face fresh.

A teaspoon of almond oil mixed with a teaspoon of *amla* juice massaged over the scalp is a valuable remedy for loss of hair, scanty growth, dandruff and premature greying.

Groundnut *(momphali)* : The oil from the groundnut can serve as a beauty aid. A teaspoon of refined groundnut oil, mixed with an equal quantity of lime juice, may be applied daily on the face before going to bed. It keeps the face fresh. Its regular use nourishes the skin and prevents acne.

OTHER FOODS

Curd *(dahi)* : Curd is considered one of the best aids to natural goods looks. It supplies the nerves and the skin with healthy ingredients and counteracts the ill-effects of exposure to the scorching sun. The bacteria in curd make the skin soft and glowing. Curd mixed with orange or lemon juice is a good face cleanser. It supplies moisture to the skin and fruit juice provides the essential vitamin C. One spoonful of juice should be mixed in one cup of curd. This should be applied to the face and neck and allowed to dry for 15 minutes. It should then be wiped off with a soft tissue and washed with water.

A mixture of oatmeal flour and yoghurt has been found effective in making the skin brighter and softer. This mixture should be kept on the face for 15 to 20 minutes and then washed off with warm water. For pimples, a paste of curd and Bengal gram flour *(besan)* should be applied on the face and then washed off.

Curd is also considered valuable in conditioning the hair. It makes the hair soft, healthy and strong. Curd should be massaged right into the scalp and then washed off. Dandruff can be removed by massaging one's hair for half an hour with curd which has been kept in the open for three days.

Honey *(shahad)* : A mixture of honey and alcohol is believed to promote the growth of hair. It is said that Japanese geisha girls, who have luxuriant hair, mix several tablespoons of honey with alcohol, and stir them together. They massage this mixture into the scalp, allow it to remain there for two hours and then shampoo it out thoroughly. It is said that regular use of this honey-alcohol mixture stimulates the hair follicles to grow into luxuriant tresses.

Milk *(dudh)* : Milk is useful as a cosmetic and as a beauty aid. A fresh lime should be squeezed in a glass of boiled milk and set for 10 minutes. It should then be applied over hands, arms, face, neck and soles at night and allowed to dry. It should be washed off with warm water in the morning. Its regular use will whiten the complexion and make the skin soft. Washing the hair with milk and egg yolk every day will promote hair growth and protect the scalp from all diseases.

CHAPTER 17

HERBS AS BEAUTY AIDS

It is generally believed that the use of cosmetics originated in China over 4,000 years ago. A lot of general information on herbs and their uses was gathered and recorded in the first 'Herbal' by the Chinese Emperor Shen Nung, in 3,000 B.C. The earliest evidence of cosmetics, however, comes from Egypt. There it was customary to bury, along with the mummyfied bodies of pharaohs and their consorts, samples of the comforts and luxuries available to them in their earthly lifetime, for use in their after-life.

Early experiments in the field of herbal cosmetics were carried out by Galen, a Greek physician who lived in the second century A.D. He discovered that vegetable oil could be mixed with water and melted beeswax, and that the resulting cream when smoothed on the skin, was cool and soothing; not only did the skin become soft but it also became supple. He had, thus, discovered what we know today as 'cold cream'.

Much progress has been made in herbal cosmetics, since Galen's time. Today there are a wide range of natural herbs which are of great cosmetic value. They can be beneficially used as beauty aids. Some of the important herbs which can be used in this manner are described here in brief.

Alfalfa : The juice of alfalfa in combination with the juices of carrot and lettuce, taken daily, will help the growth of hair to a remarkable extent. The combination of these juices is rich in elements which are particularly useful for the roots of the hair.

Camomile : The herb is a versatile beauty-aid. It is familiar weed, found in many waste lands. It possesses the properties to control acne, soothe skin irrritations and cleanse the skin of blemishes. An infusion of the leaves and flowers of this plant, fresh or dried, can be used beneficially for these purposes.

Castor *(arandi)* : The oil from castor seeds massaged over the body, before having a bath, is said to keep one's skin healthy and imparts sound sleep. This oil bath may be taken once a week. Applying castor oil over the hands and feet before going to bed keeps them soft. Its regular use as a hair oil helps the growth of hair and cures dandruff. Its regular application over the eye-brows and eye-lashes keeps them trim and improves their looks.

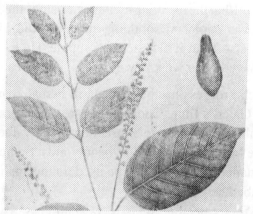

Chebulic Myrobalan is useful as a hair tonic.

Chebulic Myrobalan (*harad* or *haritaki*) : The herb is useful as a hair tonic. A paste of the fruit is boiled in coconut oil till its essence completely dissolves in the oil. This oil used regularly gives vitality to the hair. A decoction made from chebulic myrobalan is a popular hair rinse which many Indian women use to blacken grey hair.

Chicory *(Kasni)* : Chicory has been mentioned as a special skin beautifier by the ancient herbalists. A tea made from the pale blue flowers of this plant was said to give the 'plainest maid a measure of loveliness by her bright shining skin'. According to a legend, chicory got this reputation because of a beautiful woman whom the sun wished to marry. But she spurned him. On her refusal, he turned her into a wild chicory plant and ensured that her fragile flowers would be forever turned towards him, whenever he was in the sky, from dawn till dusk. No one knows whether this legend arose before chicory had earned its name as a complexion improving drink, or after. But the flowers used for making a tea to drink seem to give the skin a healthy glow.

Cinnamon *(dalchini)* : A paste of cinnamon powder prepared with a few drops of fresh lime juice can be applied over pimples and blackheads with beneficial results. The oil extract of cinnamon can be used for massage. It soothes sunburnt skins.

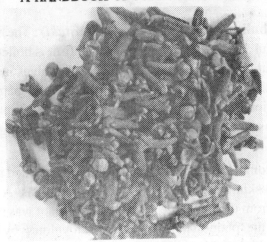

Clove soothes eruptions and rashes on the skin.

Clove *(laung)* : This herb has powerful antiseptic properties. It heals and soothes eruptions and rashes on the skin. It is used in medicated creams. It also helps to decrease infection in teeth and freshes the breath.

Euphorbia *(lal dudhi)* : The milky juice of this plant is useful in promoting hair growth. It should be applied to the scalp for this purpose.

Fennel *(saunf)* : This herbs exercises a cleansing effect on the skin especially for deep-pore cleansing. It can be used beneficially in water while steaming the face. It has also been used in herbal hair rinses.

Henna *(mehndi)* : Henna can be used beneficially as a treatment for falling of hair and other hair problems such as dandruff, premature greying and alopecia or patchy baldness. Mustard oil boiled with henna leaves promotes healthy growth of hair. The procedure for preparing this oil has been explained in Chapter 11 on Hair Disorders.

The paste of henna leaves boiled in coconut oil to get a darkish oil, can be used as a hair dye to blacken grey hair. The paste itself can be applied to the hair and washed off after a few hours to dye the grey hair.

Apart from colouring the hair, it is a very good conditioner. Chemical dyes can in fact damage the hair structure, but henna protects it. It also adds beauty, body and bounce to the hair, leaving it supple, shiny and easy to manage.

Henna is also a good cleanser and does not destroy the acidic nature of the scalp. Its paste mixed with lemon juice, egg and yoghurt, is one of the best methods of cleaning and conditioning the hair. It also promotes hair growth and a healthy scalp and acts as an anti-dandruff agent.

Indian Sarsaparilla *(magarbu anantma)* : A decoction of sarsaparilla root used as a hair wash is said to promote hair growth. The herb contains the important hair-growing hormone alongwith other constituents.

Indian Senna *(bhumiari)* : A paste of the dried leaves made with vinegar can be used for certain skin diseases. The paste is also useful for removing pimples.

Indian Spikenard *(jatamansi)* : *Jatamansi* is well-known as a hair tonic. It is an important ingredient of many hair washes and hair oils.

Margosa *(neem)* : The leaves of the margosa tree are valuable in hair disorders. If the hair has been falling or has ceased to grow, it should be washed with a decoction of neem leaves. This will stop the hair from falling

127

and will stabilize its blackness. It will also lengthen the hair and kill lice and other infesting insects on the scalp.

Marigold *(saldbargh* or *zergul)* : An infusion of marigold petals, applied as a lotion provides an ideal balancer of an over-oily skin and is good for all complexions.

Rose *(gulab-ke-phul)* : This flower has a luxurious aroma and has been in use from ancient times. The petals of this flower are used for making rose water, which forms an ideal base for skin tonics. It helps to soften coarse skin. It is used in lotions and creams, for its soothing and gentle action.

Rosemary *(rusmari)* : The herbs rosemary is beneficial in the treatment of hair disorders. Shampoo and hair lotions containing pure extract of this herb, bring new life to the scalp and hair while preventing dandruff and premature baldness. A simple home-made lotion from leafy rosemary branches can be prepared by simmering them in water for 30 minutes. This should then be strained and allowed to cool. This lotion can be poured over the hair as a final rinse.

Sage *(salvia)* : The herb is considered useful in preventing greying of hair. It is said to bring colour back to greying hair when it is included in hair tonics.

Sandalwood *(chandan)* : It has a powerful antiseptic and germicidal effect. An emulsion or a paste of the wood is a cooling dressing in inflammatory and eruptive conditions of the skin. The oil of sandalwood, mixed with twice its quantity of mustard oil, can be used beneficially for removing pimples. In summer, the regular application of sandalwood paste on the body, has a refreshing effect, which heals any tiny infected spots.

Saussurea *(kuth)* : The herb is useful in hair disorders. It is said to have the power to prevent premature greying of the hair. Dried and powdered roots can be used beneficially as a hair wash.

DR. BAKHRU'S
BESTSELLERS WITH JAICO

• **A Complete Handbook of Nature Cure** (Revised & Enlarged Edition)

This revised and enlarged handbook is a most comprehensive family guide to health the natural way. Author makes a compelling case, for treating diseases through natural methods which rely on natural foods, natural elements, yoga and observance of other laws of nature. This well illustrated book is no doubt beneficial for those who desire good health through the use of natural remedies. The book also contains numerous food charts to enable the readers to plan their daily diet for good health.

In view of its valuable contents, this book has been awarded first prize under the category Primer on Naturopathy For Healthy Living by the jury of judges. This prize was given at "Book Prize Award Scheme" for the year 1997-1998 instituted by the National Institute of Naturopathy, an autonomous body under Government of India, Ministry of Health and Family Welfare.

• **Diet Cure for Common Ailments**

This book covers the whole gamut of ailments which can be cured merely by proper food habits and regulation of one's life, without recourse to medicinal treatment. The book is based on the theories and fundamentals of Nature Cure that go to preserve health and vitality and regain these when lost. It is a useful guide to those who wish to treat themselves through this system at home.

• **Nature Cure For Children**

This book gives all essential tips you require to put your "little one" at ease. It is an alternative way out to treat your child and keep the doctor at bay. It helps you discover:
— What to do when worms infest your child's tummy
— What to do when lice swarm all over your child's head
— How to give a hot water enema
— How to apply mud packs
— How to give a massage and ..... a lot more.

• Healing Through Natural Foods

This book lays great stress on the diet as the best and safest form of alternative medicines. Based on the latest scientific researches, it shows that foods affect cellular behaviour, which may lead to health or diseases. It also describes in some details preventive and healing powers of the specific foods in specific diseases by virtue of miracle drugs contained in them.

• Naturopathy For Longevity

The book deals with diseases commonly prevalent in the elderly and prescribes time-tested nature cure methods for their treatment. It contains invaluable nature cure methods which if practised sincerely can work miracles for problems related with ageing viz. poor health, loss of functions, slower mental faculties and development of other frightening diseases.

• Indian Spices And Condiments As Natural Healers

Spices and condiments are one of the most important forms of natural foods. Besides culinary uses, they have been used in indigenous system of medicine as natural healers since ancient times. They thus form part of our heritage healing. This book describes in great detail the medicinal virtues of different specific spices and condiments, and their usefulness in the treatment of various common ailments. This information can serve as a guide to the readers to solve their common health problems through the use of specific spices and condiments, besides adopting a well-balanced natural diet.

Dear Booklover,

Thank you very much for buying this book. We hope that you have enjoyed reading it. In our endeavor to keep you informed about our new releases, please do email the following information to jaicopub@vsnl.com:

Title(s)with J number(s): ....

....

Bookstore: ....

City: ....

Your Name: ....

Email Address: ....

Subjects of Interest (Fiction/Non-Fiction/Business/Engineering):

Other Comments: ....

Please do visit our website www.jaicobooks.com for more information regarding our titles.